WEIGHT
LOSS
SURGERY

WEIGHT LOSS SURGERY

Is It Right For You?

MERLE CANTOR GOLDBERG, LCSW
WILLIAM Y. MARCUS, MD
& GEORGE COWAN, JR., MD

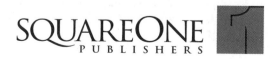
SQUAREONE
PUBLISHERS

COVER DESIGNER: Phaedra Mastrocola and Jeannie Tudor
EDITOR: Carol A. Rosenberg
TYPESETTER: Gary A. Rosenberg

The information and advice contained in this book are based upon the research and
the personal and professional experiences of the authors. They are not intended as a
substitute for consulting with a health-care professional. The publisher and authors
are not responsible for any adverse effects or consequences resulting from the use of
any of the suggestions, preparations, or procedures discussed in this book. All matters pertaining to your physical health should be supervised by a health-care professional. It is a sign of wisdom, not cowardice, to seek a second or third opinion.

Names have been changes to protect the privacy of the individuals who shared their
personal stories with the authors.

Square One Publishers
115 Herricks Road
Garden City Park, NY 11040
(516) 535-2010 • (877) 900-BOOK
www.squareonepublishers.com

Library of Congress Cataloging-in-Publication Data

Cantor Goldberg, Merle.
  Weight-loss surgery : is it right for you? / Merle Cantor Goldberg,
William Y. Marcus, George Cowan, Jr.
    p. cm.
  Includes bibliographical references and index.
  ISBN 0-7570-0145-9 (pbk.)
  1. Obesity—Surgery. 2. Gastrointestinal system—Surgery. 3. Weight loss.
I. Marcus, William Y. II. Cowan, George. III. Title.
  RD540.C35   2006
  617.4'3—dc22
                                                              2005034917

Printed in the United States of America

10   9   8   7   6   5   4   3   2   1

CONTENTS

A Word About Gender, vii

Acknowledgments, ix

Preface, xi

Introduction, 1

PART ONE
DECIDING IF WEIGHT-LOSS SURGERY IS RIGHT FOR YOU

1. Know Your Enemy—Obesity and Obesity-Related Health Conditions, 5
2. Do You Qualify for Surgery?, 19
3. Which Option Is Right for You?, 35
4. Making and Sharing Your Decision, 55

PART TWO
YOUR JOURNEY FROM PRESURGERY TO RECOVERY

5. Support—An Essential Element, 75
6. Your First Medical Appointment and Presurgical Tests, 93
7. The Days Before and the Day of Surgery, 111
8. What to Expect Immediately After Surgery, 131
9. Your Arrival Home and the First Six Months, 155

PART THREE
YOUR FUTURE—
THIN AND HEALTHY FOR LIFE

10. Six Months and Beyond, 185

11. Your Most Important Relationship—The One You Have With Yourself, 197

12. A Second Chance—Your Relationships With Others, 219

PART FOUR
FOR FRIENDS AND FAMILY

13. How You Can Make a Difference Before Surgery, 233

14. After Surgery, You Are Essential, 243

Conclusion, 259

Glossary, 261

Resources, 267

References, 269

About the Authors, 271

Index, 273

*To all of our patients with morbid obesity,
past and present, for whom all of our efforts are made.*

*While working for them and with them during their journey
toward improved health, we have learned much.*

$\mathcal{A}$ WORD
ABOUT GENDER

To avoid awkward phrasing within sentences, the publisher has chosen to alternate the use of male and female pronouns according to chapter. Therefore, odd-numbered chapters use male pronouns, while even-numbered chapters employ female pronouns, to give acknowledgment to medical personnel and surgical candidates of both genders.

$\mathcal{A}$CKNOWLEDGMENTS

Weight-loss surgery is a serious and complicated procedure that is performed on a high-risk population. It requires the ongoing involvement of a talented and dedicated health-care team. Every aspect of this surgery, both before and after, requires demanding skills, continuing education, and, most of all, long-haul dedication. Therefore, we would like to acknowledge all the skilled surgeons, nurses, staff members, and mental-health specialists who put forth their best efforts to ensure the health and well-being of every person who chooses to undergo weight-loss surgery.

We would also like to thank our colleagues for their collaboration in our ongoing work to improve the lives of people with morbid obesity—Dr. Barry Greene; program directors Jeanne Ferber, Julia Hernandez, and Alfreda Hill Wilkerson; Adrienne Ressler; Sandy Arioli; Barbara Metzger; Dr. Don Revis; Dr. Francis Chiamonte; Dr. Michael Vincent; Dr. Emmett (Rick) Bishop; Dr. Jarol Boan; and Dr. Cathy Reto.

We would also like to thank our patients for openly and courageously sharing their lives and their stories with us. A special thanks to Bob, as well as to Wendy, Susan, Kathy, Donna, Mike, Dennis, Patti, Larry, Michelle, Rick, Beth, Kristi, Marion, and all the other very special patients who have enriched our book, but even more important, our lives.

Merle Goldberg wishes to acknowledge her family for their patience, love, and support—first and foremost, her extraordinary husband, Dr. Walter Goozh, and very special daughter, Stephanie Goozh; Andrew and Diane Speyrer; Julian and Justin Astley; Cynthia and Chris Brown; Jennifer Bergmann; Dr. Jerry and Wendy Santoro; Eric Santoro and Jennifer Jordan; Craig Santoro; Joanne and Nate Sternberg; and Mom-mom. Her most special thanks to her father, Col. Stanley L. Cantor, and mother, Alberta Gottfried Cantor, who taught her that anything is possible.

Dr. George Cowan, Jr., wishes to acknowledge his family's loving support—most important his wife, Anne; his son Scot Cowan and his wife, Michelle; his son G. S. Marshall Cowan III and his wife, Saadia; his daughter, Katie Sentilles, and her husband, Shawn; his grandchildren, Sabrina, Claire Anne, Quinn, Francie, and his namesake George; and his mother, Beatrice Cowan.

$\mathscr{P}$REFACE

lthough it was many years ago, I recall that the day had been an extraordinarily long one. I'd started seeing patients at 7:30 that morning, and eleven hours later, I was tired and hungry. But there I was in the hospital basement, getting ready to give a lecture on emotional eating. I leaned against the doorpost for support and peered into the cavernous room. It was filled to overflowing with the 250-plus members of the hospital's weight-loss-surgery support group.

The atmosphere in the room was charged—lively, supportive, and expectant. Most people moved around freely, while others clustered in small groups. A few people seemed aloof, perhaps somewhat apprehensive. (I later learned that these were the "pre-op" people, new to the group and to the prospect of undergoing weight-loss surgery.)

The room quieted down as the program director and patient leader began the meeting. (My talk would come during the second half of the meeting.) A few courageous group members, those who had undergone the surgery, rose to share their stories of success. This time, I was not the speech-giver but the listener, and I listened intently. I was drawn in by what they said and touched in a way that surprised me. I found myself moved by the honest display of emotions, by the climate of mutual support, and, most of all, by the courage these people exhibited.

The intensity of their feelings came through as they spoke about the positive changes in their family lives after their weight loss: *My grandson can get his little arms around me for a hug! . . . My kids aren't ashamed of me anymore and don't ask me to drop them off down the block from their destination.* They also talked about their improved body images and better health: *I can finally buy off-the-rack clothing! . . . I've lost eighty-five pounds, and, what do you know, I do have a collarbone! . . . My doctor says that my diabetes has greatly improved. . . . I can walk a flight of stairs without running out of breath.* They also touched upon work-related issues: *I finally got the promotion I had waited for for so long. Doesn't my boss know it's the same me?* And, as the first half of the meeting died down, they spoke of the simple everyday things that so many of us take for granted: *I don't have to stay at home to watch movies anymore—I can fit in the seats at the theater! . . . I can walk around comfortably in public without being ridiculed or stared at.*

Over the next few weeks, I could not get the group out of my mind. I wanted to learn more about morbid obesity and its emotional ramifications and the surgery to correct it. The knowledge I sought as a result of that first meeting long ago became an important part of my practice and my life.

Morbid obesity is one of America's most significant health problems. Most of us are aware of the increased health risks that accompany obesity—high blood pressure, heart disease, diabetes, certain cancers, back and joint problems, sleep apnea, breathing problems, skin disorders, and so on. Being obese also dramatically increases the risk of death. Unfortunately, medical problems are only a small part of the picture. For people who are obese, weight affects every area of their lives—physical, psychological, social, and economic. Being overweight may indeed affect every one of their relationships—business and personal. Weight-related issues remain a constant source of anguish and social pressure, and, to some degree, they determine the outcome of virtually every interaction and relationship.

So many obese people spend their lives battling their weight and obesity-related problems—they try diet, behavior modification, weight-loss pills, and so on—unfortunately, without long-term success. This is why increasing numbers of morbidly obese people are turning to weight-loss surgery as a long-term solution.

Along with the growing interest in this surgery has come an increasing amount of media coverage. Some of this coverage has been accurate and thought-provoking. Other coverage has been sensationalized, presenting an incomplete or inaccurate picture. That's why my coauthors and I have written this book. It's here to dispel misconceptions and to clarify the truth. It's here to provide people who are contemplating weight-loss surgery with the information and support they need to face their upcoming journey with courage.

We are delighted to be putting our years of experience as internationally recognized weight-loss-surgery experts, as well as the experiences of thousands of our patients, to work for our readers. It is our intention to be partners in their health and well-being and to provide some insight into the world of the weight-loss-surgery health-care team. For those who choose to undergo the surgery, we hope that they find support in these pages as they change—not only externally, but also internally.

Perhaps the words of one of our patients sums up the best reason for writing this book: "Before the surgery, I thought I was afraid to die. What I realized after the surgery was that I had really been afraid to live. Doctor, you have given me back my life."

—Merle Cantor Goldberg, LCSW

$\mathcal{I}$NTRODUCTION

f you've picked up this book, chances are you are among the nearly 16 million Americans who are overweight enough to be candidates for weight-loss surgery, also called *bariatric surgery*. You are concerned about your health, and you want to do something to improve it. You are wise to be alarmed, since more than 300,000 deaths each year in this country stem from obesity and its related health conditions.

Perhaps you are one of the nearly 200,000 Americans who have decided to have weight-loss surgery this year, and you're looking for some reliable information. Or maybe you haven't yet made a decision, and you're in need of some guidance. Or perhaps your spouse, family member, or friend is preparing to have the surgery, and you want to know more about what's involved and how you can help. Or maybe you've already had the surgery and simply want a better idea of what to expect in the coming months.

No matter which category you fall into, this book is for you. It is your comprehensive reference guide to weight-loss surgery and its short-term and long-term effects. It will guide you through the entire process—from the earliest inklings of contemplating surgery and the decision-making process to the surgery itself, recovery from the surgery, and long-term issues.

Part One of *Weight-Loss Surgery: Is It Right For You?* begins with the key issue of deciding if weight-loss surgery is a good choice for you. This surgery is a serious and complicated medical procedure, and the decision to take this step is quite complex and personal. Since it has the potential to alter every aspect of your health and life, this is one of the most important decisions you'll ever make. It is essential to learn all you can in order to make the best decision. To help with your decision, this part defines the levels of obesity, from morbid obesity to end-stage obesity syndrome, as well as many of the health conditions that can accompany serious weight problems. Next, it discusses the qualifications for weight-loss surgery—both physical and emotional. Then, it details the various types of weight-loss surgery you might have available to you, including the pros and cons of each. The final chapter in this part takes you through the process of choosing a surgeon and sharing your final decision with the people closest to you.

Part Two deals with what happens after you've made your decision to have the surgery. It explains why it's necessary to have a support system in place and where you can look for help. Then, you'll find out what happens at your very first medical appointment. You'll also learn what presurgical tests are required, how to prepare for surgery, what happens during the surgery itself, and what to expect at various stages of recovery. You'll also receive some guidance on diet and exercise.

In Part Three, every aspect of your "second chance" is covered, including matters concerning your existing relationships, dating, and marriage. You'll learn how to deal with the changes that can and will occur in your life and your relationships. Most important, you'll get an up-close look at your most intimate relationship—the one you have with yourself. It's no secret that massive weight loss poses challenges to both your body image and self-image. This part will help guide you through those changes. If you've already had the surgery, you can skip directly to this part. It can help clarify or address any difficulties you may be experiencing, as well as provide you with new and creative ideas to add to your existing program as you journey toward "forever health."

The support and understanding of your loved ones are essential elements in surgical success and long-term health. Therefore, Part Four is written specifically for those people who know someone who plans to have weight-loss surgery and want to understand the procedure and help in any way they can. It's full of advice to help everyone make a smooth transition, before and after surgery.

Weight-loss surgery isn't an easy, magical process where weight falls off and everyone lives happily ever after. While the results *are* dramatic, weight-loss surgery is a long, winding, and continually challenging road that involves much knowledge and a strong commitment. There may be some bumps along the way and a small risk of life-threatening complications. The full story is in this book, not just the wealth of good news but *all* of the news. Have a safe and successful journey.

PART ONE

*Deciding If
Weight-Loss Surgery
Is Right for You*

CHAPTER 1

*K*NOW YOUR ENEMY
Obesity and Obesity–Related Health Conditions

Chances are you've been living with obesity and its related conditions, often referred to as *comorbidities,* for many years. Perhaps you've never given much thought to the medical terms and definitions that apply to your condition. Now, however, you are seeking answers and want to gather as much information as possible before making the decision to have weight-loss surgery. Being familiar with some of the medical terms you may come across during your search will help you better understand your choices. Therefore, this chapter begins by defining the term *obesity* in general. It then goes on to explain more serious forms of obesity, including morbid obesity and super-morbid obesity. Next, it discusses various obesity comorbidities, such as type-2 diabetes, heart disease, breathing difficulties, sleep apnea, and high blood pressure, which weight-loss surgery can usually help improve or correct.

WHAT IS OBESITY?

To win a battle, you must first know your enemy. In this case, understanding how obesity is defined is a first step toward conquering this condition. So, let's begin with a detailed definition: *Obesity is a lifelong, progressive, life-threatening, genetically related disease of excessive fat storage with five major groups of comorbidities—medical, physical, psychological, social, and economic.* That's a bit of a mouthful, isn't it? Let's take a look at each part of the definition to better understand what this disease is really all about.

Unlike an episode of the flu or chickenpox, obesity is a *lifelong* condition. It often begins in childhood, and if successful long-term steps aren't taken to treat it, it will continue for the life of the obese person. The fact that it is not a fleeting condition becomes quite important when considering possible treatments. A treatment that works for only a few months, or even for a year or two, is not the answer. Short-term treatments have no real lasting value. Most diets, medications, ear-stapling procedures, acupuncture sessions, hypnosis, herbal extracts, and so on are short-term treatments. It's important for people, especially obese people, to understand that short-term treatments can't resolve a lifelong condition such as obesity.

Obesity is also a *progressive* condition. In other words, an obese person's weight generally increases by a half pound to twenty-five pounds per year, depending upon various factors. As weight increases, the risk of developing life-threatening and/or life-altering comorbidities also increases. When an obese person has one or more of these conditions and others begin to develop, obesity can become *life threatening*.

Millions of years of evolution, as well as numerous scientific studies, show that *genetics* is one of the causes of obesity and that being obese is *not* just a matter of poor willpower. Beneath our basic survival instincts, such as our need to eat, lies a powerful inheritance from our ancestors—our genes. These genes, which are part of every one of our bodies' cells, largely make us what we are. There is evidence that certain genes cause obesity. Research is ongoing to identify the genes responsible and how best to deal with them.

That brings us to the last word in our definition: *disease*. Are you surprised that obesity is a disease? The U.S. government and the World Health Organization (WHO) recognize obesity as a disease, and as such, it is listed in the International Classification of Diseases, a list of codes for recognized diseases, under number 278.0. This list is used every day, in one way or another, in the practice of medicine.

So there you have it. *Obesity is a lifelong, progressive, life-threatening, genetically related disease of excessive fat storage with five major groups of comorbidities.* A little later in the chapter, we'll take a close look at several of the comorbidities, some of which may be more familiar to you than others. But first, to fully understand what obesity is, let's review the meaning of the terms *morbid obesity, super-morbid obesity,* and *end-stage obesity syndrome.*

Morbid Obesity

Obesity becomes regarded as morbid, or disease-causing, when it reaches the point of significantly increasing the risk of developing one or more serious diseases, or comorbidities. Morbid obesity is typically defined as being 100 pounds or more over ideal body weight, having a body mass index

(BMI) of 35 to 39.9 with comorbidities, or a BMI of 40 or higher without comorbidities. These are usually the levels at which someone may qualify for weight-loss surgery. (See Chapters 2 and 4 for a discussion of BMI and ideal body weight, respectively.) Morbid obesity is also listed in the International Classification of Diseases. Its classification number is 278.01.

Super-Morbid Obesity

An even more severe form of morbid obesity is super-morbid obesity. This is defined as being 2.25 times the ideal weight for height and frame size according to the standardized height-weight tables used by many insurance companies. (For example, according to such tables, the average ideal weight for a medium-framed woman who is 5'4" is 140 pounds. Two and a quarter times this average ideal weight is 315 pounds.) Many experts also describe people with a BMI of 50 or higher as having super-morbid obesity. People who have reached such weights have a higher risk of disease and death than those who are morbidly obese. Some people with super-morbid obesity are too ill to undergo any type of surgery, much less weight-loss surgery, especially in the case of end-stage obesity syndrome (ESOS), discussed next.

End-Stage Obesity Syndrome (ESOS)

When a morbidly obese or super-morbidly obese person's condition reaches the point of organ failure, the condition is termed *end-stage obesity syndrome* (ESOS). This syndrome was first described by coauthor Dr. Cowan in August 1994, at a conference of the International Association for the Study of Obesity in Toronto, Canada. In medical terminology, the term *end-stage* means "occurring in the final stages of a terminal disease." In ESOS, a person is experiencing failure of one or more organ systems. Without treatment, he is likely to die within weeks or months. The first step in treating someone with ESOS is to get the organ failure under control. This includes putting the person on an extremely strict weight-loss program, and if enough weight is lost, he may then become a candidate for weight-loss surgery.

In these cases, treatment is long term and high risk. Also, the cost can be very high, sometimes amounting to hundreds of thousands of dollars. The fact that most people with ESOS have short lives remaining without treatment compounds the problem. However, we have successfully treated a large majority of our ESOS patients. The lesson we've learned from our work in this area, however, is that obese people need effective treatment *well before* they develop ESOS.

MEDICAL CONDITIONS ASSOCIATED WITH OBESITY

In this book, the term *comorbidity* describes a group of medical and physical illnesses, as well as psychological, social, and economic conditions, that often occur alongside, or get worse with, obesity. You are probably already aware of many of the psychological, social, and economic drawbacks that often accompany obesity. We'll touch upon these non-medical-related drawbacks in our discussions throughout this book. Meanwhile, the following list, which you'll note is quite long, sets forth the most common medical comorbidities, some of which are more serious than others. The sections to follow discuss several of these issues.

- Anxiety disorder
- Body odor (severe)
- Bone, joint, and/or muscle pain, including in the neck, back, hips, legs, knees, ankles, and/or feet
- Breathing difficulties, including chronic wheezing
- Bronchitis, chronic
- Cancer
- Cervical disk disease
- Coronary artery disease (CAD)
- Depression
- Dermatitis
- Diabetes, type-2
- Enlarged liver
- Exertion difficulties
- Gallbladder disease
- Gastritis, chronic
- Gout
- Heart problems
- Heel spurs
- Hiatus hernia
- High levels of "bad" fat in the blood
- Hirsutism (excess facial and body hair)
- Hypertension (high blood pressure)
- Infertility
- Leg ulcers (venous stasis)
- Liver disease (cirrhosis)
- Lumbar disk disease
- Malaise, general
- Menstrual irregularities
- Obesity-hypoventilation syndrome
- Osteoarthritis and other forms of arthritis
- Pseudotumor cerebri (fluid pressure on the brain)
- Pulmonary embolus (blockage of an artery in the lungs)
- Renal (kidney) disease
- Restless leg syndrome
- Sleep apnea
- Thrombosis, deep venous
- Urinary stress incontinence
- Varicose veins
- Walking difficulties
- Weakness

Breathing Difficulties

Many morbidly obese people experience difficulty breathing with little exertion. For example, simply climbing a half of a flight of stairs can result in shortness of breath and a pounding heart. Even at rest, the lungs of a morbidly obese person cannot take as much air into the body as can the lungs of an average-weight person. This is usually because the excess fat interferes with the full expansion of the chest during inhalation. Fortunately, for this reason shortness of breath with exertion resolves for most people following massive weight loss.

Bone, Joint, and/or Muscle Pains

Bone, joint, and/or muscle pains can become such a normal part of an obese person's daily life that he actually fails to mention these symptoms on health-history questionnaires. Even some obese people who have arthritis fail to mention their aches and pains. For others, however, the pain is so excruciating and debilitating that it is the first problem they mention.

Excess weight placed on the bones and joints can cause many serious physical disabilities, especially of the feet, ankles, knees, hips, and lower back. Serious back problems can occur when the curve of the lower back becomes exaggerated due to stretched-out abdominal muscles and tightened back muscles resulting from the effects of obesity and inactivity. This exaggerated curve often leads to back strain, slipped lumbar or cervical disks, and arthritis.

Many morbidly obese people are advised by their physicians to lose weight before undergoing hip, back, or knee surgery due to the higher risks involved. In our experience, nearly every patient with bone, joint, and/or muscle pain experiences less pain after shedding a substantial amount of weight. In fact, many of our patients who were considering knee, hip, or back surgery concluded that it was unnecessary at their reduced weights.

Cancer

Research shows that obese women tend to develop breast cancer three times more often than their non-obese counterparts. Moreover, morbidly obese women are three times more likely to develop ovarian cancer and five times more likely to develop endometrial cancer than non-obese women. Similarly, morbidly obese men have a three times greater chance of developing prostate cancer than non-obese men. There seems to be a few reasons for this.

Research by Dr. Cowan and colleagues at the University of Tennessee found that obese people have lower levels of antioxidants in their bodies than non-obese people. As you may already know, antioxidants are needed to protect the body's cells, including DNA, from damage by destructive free-radical molecules. The low levels of antioxidants found in these individuals seemed to result in more DNA damage than an average-weight person would normally experience. Since DNA damage can lead to cancer, as well as to other diseases, low levels of antioxidants are linked to an increased cancer risk. Also, cancer-causing substances, known as *carcinogens,* some of which are found in the foods we eat, dissolve better in fat than in water. Therefore, with their greater food intake and their excess body fat, morbidly obese people end up absorbing and storing more cancer-causing substances. This, coupled with fewer antioxidants, explains the increased cancer risk quite clearly.

Massive weight loss should, and thus far appears to, reduce the increased risk of developing cancer associated with morbid obesity.

Diabetes

Dr. Cowan's patient Diana complained of frequent urination, constant thirst, and recurring bladder infections. It was pretty clear from these symptoms that Diana had diabetes mellitus, and tests confirmed it. However, like many morbidly obese patients, Diana was unaware that she had this condition.

An average of 14 to 18 percent of morbidly obese people have diabetes mellitus. Of these, more than 96 percent have type-2 diabetes, formerly called *adult-onset diabetes.* This condition can often be treated with medication and dietary changes. Substantial weight loss, however, can actually cure a person of type-2 diabetes. In fact, more than 90 percent of our patients who had type-2 diabetes prior to weight-loss surgery no longer had it after their significant weight loss.

Enlarged Liver (Hepatomegaly)

We have found that more than 95 percent of obese people have some type of liver abnormality, usually resulting in a liver that is beyond its normal size. In liver samples taken from every 100 morbidly obese patients, all but five are usually abnormal. About one-third has severe amounts of fat in the liver, one-third has moderate amounts, and one-third has mild amounts. A number of pateints also have scarring of the liver, as found in cirrhosis. According to our findings, most of the livers of our morbidly obese patients seem to gradually get smaller and appear healthier as excess fat is lost.

Gallbladder Disease

Gallstones form when cholesterol levels in the gallbladder become so concentrated that the cholesterol cannot stay dissolved in the bile and begins to form crystals. These crystals attract even more cholesterol and grow rapidly into gallstones. Once gallstones have formed, a person becomes at risk for cholecystitis, inflammation of the gallbladder.

A gallbladder "attack" occurs when a small stone blocks the flow of bile while it passes through the common bile duct into the intestines, often causing jaundice—yellowing of the skin, eyes, and body fluids—and pain, usually in the right upper abdomen. Gallbladder bile is also more likely to become infected when gallstones are present, resulting in inflammation and fever, as well as other symptoms and risks.

Once stones have formed in the gallbladder, they will almost always keep forming there. Therefore, to prevent future gallbladder attacks, the gallbladder needs to be removed. In fact, about one-third of morbidly obese people will have their gallbladders removed at some point in their lives.

It's also important to note that, after large amounts of weight loss for any reason, including diet, medications, or surgery, there will be a greater concentration of cholesterol in the bile due to the breakdown of fat, and gallstones are more likely to form. Therefore, as discussed in Chapter 3, some surgeons recommend gallbladder removal during weight-loss surgery.

Heart Problems and Coronary Artery Disease (CAD)

Picture two people lined up to run fifty yards. Both are about the same height, but one of them is morbidly obese while the other is of average weight. They begin running, but the obese person stops after about twenty to thirty steps, breathless. Meanwhile, the non-obese person is able to complete the fifty yards. The morbidly obese person's heart just couldn't handle the strain. Even at rest, that person's heart had one-and-a-half to two times more blood to pump per minute than the non-obese person's heart due to his larger size. So, when they began to run, the obese person's already overworked heart had trouble increasing its pumping capacity. Having coronary artery disease (CAD)—a disease in which the arteries that supply blood to the heart muscles are narrowed—makes this problem even worse. An obese person with CAD would find it even more difficult, if not impossible, to run or jog. Obesity is responsible for the 58 to 70 percent of Americans who develop severe CAD—the primary cause of many of the 300,000 obesity-related deaths that occur each year in this country.

In one study, Dr. Cowan performed exercise tests on sixty-two of his patients using a gamma camera, a medical imaging device, to measure the amount of blood the heart pumps per beat as well as to study the movement of the walls of the heart. The result of this study was shocking. Most of the patients had some type of abnormality. Two-thirds were so abnormal that the team cardiologist recommended further studies. Later, most of the patients, especially those whose heart studies looked the worst before surgery, experienced improvement six or more months after their massive weight loss.

Hiatus Hernia

On the history section of her health questionnaire, Gina circled the following complaints: heartburn; pain behind the breastbone; burp often; occasional acid-tasting liquid in mouth; and swallowed food sometimes "sticks." From these responses, it was almost certain Gina had a hiatus hernia.

The word *hiatus* is a technical term for *opening*. In this case, the opening we're talking about is the *esophageal hiatus* of the diaphragm—in other words, the point at which the esophagus, the tube that carries food to the stomach, passes through the diaphragm. A hiatus hernia develops when the opening becomes abnormally widened due to the higher pressure in an obese person's abdomen, thereby allowing the upper part of the stomach to move through the opening meant only for the esophagus. When a person with a hiatus hernia coughs, sneezes, or strains, the pressure in the abdomen pushes the upper stomach up through the hiatus in the diaphragm into the chest. Once the stomach has moved out of its normal location into the chest, the valve at the lower end of the esophagus stops working and allows acid from the stomach to run upward into the esophagus. The bitter, acidic, clear liquid from the stomach may run right up into the mouth; this is called *waterbrash*.

The lining of the esophagus is not made to resist acid the way the stomach lining does. Therefore, when acid enters the esophagus, there is a burning felt in the upper abdomen or middle of the chest, called *heartburn*, which can often be quite painful. The irritation caused by the acid makes the lining of the esophagus swell and become somewhat narrowed with spasms, causing food to sometimes "hang up" for a little while soon after it is swallowed. It can also cause swallowed air to be burped back up. Nausea and vomiting may also occur. As discussed in Chapter 4, this condition usually improves after weight-loss surgery, but it can be repaired during weight-loss surgery if the surgeon feels it is necessary.

High Levels of "Bad" Fat in the Blood

In most cases, people who are obese have high levels of low-density lipo-proteins (LDLs), or "bad" cholesterol, and low levels of high-density lipoproteins (HDLs), or "good" cholesterol. Moreover, they usually have high levels of triglycerides, which make up about ninety-eight percent of the dietary fat we consume. Quite often, presumably because of his higher dietary-fat intake, an obese person's triglyceride levels will be well above normal. After many years, a pattern of high levels of "bad" cholesterol and triglycerides and low levels of "good" cholesterol can lead to various diseases of the blood vessels and, ultimately, heart disease.

The effects of blood vessel disease are often fatal, especially in obese individuals. In fact, it is one of the main contributors to the 300,000 deaths each year associated with obesity in this country.

Research by Dr. Cowan and others at the University of Tennessee has shown that, after significant weight loss, the levels of "good" fat among other levels increase at least slightly while the levels of "bad" fat, including the triglycerides, usually decrease to normal levels without any of the commonly prescribed medications for this condition.

Hirsutism (Excess Facial and Body Hair)

Many women who are morbidly obese have male-pattern hair growth on their face, arms, and abdomen. This condition, known as *hirsutism*, is frequently associated with excess blood levels of the male hormone testosterone, which is brought on by obesity. Along with the normal changes that occur in the levels of sex hormones as a result of weight loss, these abnormal hair patterns often improve within eighteen months or so after weight-loss surgery.

Hypertension (High Blood Pressure)

At their initial appointment, more than half of the morbidly obese patients we see are on medication for hypertension. Without losing weight and keeping it off, these people will probably need to take medication for the rest of their lives. Some of them are actually on several types of medication and still have difficulty controlling their blood pressure. Uncontrolled or poorly controlled hypertension can lead to heart attacks, stroke, and even kidney damage.

After the significant weight loss that usually follows surgery, the blood pressure readings of a large percentage of patients (80 percent in our practice) return to normal without the need for antihypertensive drugs. Most other practices have reported an improvement in at least 60 percent of their patients.

Infertility and Menstrual Irregularities

Having too much or even too little body fat can result in infertility—the inability to conceive despite trying for at least a year. One main cause of this body-fat-related infertility is due to complex changes in hormone levels that prevent the egg from leaving the ovary and passing down the Fallopian tube into the uterus where it can be fertilized. For similar reasons, obese women often have irregular, absent, or painful menstrual periods.

After some substantial weight loss, menstrual irregularity and the chances of becoming pregnant improve. However, we advise our patients to wait at least two years before attempting to get pregnant. By this time, most of the weight loss has occurred and the body's nutritional status begins to stabilize. Prior to that time, the relatively rapid weight loss will put a major strain on the nutritional demands of a growing fetus. For more information on weight-loss surgery and pregnancy, see the inset "Wait to Become Pregnant" on page 158 in Chapter 9.

Pseudotumor Cerebri (Fluid Pressure on the Brain)

Pseudotumor cerebri—a false, or pseudo, tumor of the brain—is a very rare condition that is encountered most frequently in morbidly obese people, for reasons that are not yet understood. In this condition, there is increased pressure in spinal fluid and in the fluid surrounding the brain. This condition can cause severe headaches and seriously affect one's eyesight, sometimes permanently.

Five out of six of our patients with this condition were cured of this disorder following massive weight loss. Physicians in other weight-loss centers have also reported improvement following marked weight loss in their patients with this condition.

Sleep Apnea

Joan's story was typical of someone who suffers from sleep apnea, a condition in which a person stops breathing during sleep. During our consultation, Joan complained of frequently falling asleep while talking and sometimes even while driving because she felt so exhausted. She explained that she would wake up several times during the night, sometimes to use the bathroom and other times with the sensation that she was choking. She tossed and turned so much in her sleep that her sheets and blankets were "all over the place." She was told that she snored very loudly and that sometimes she seemed to stop breathing in her sleep. Joan said she felt even more tired in the mornings than when she went to bed. Aside from her sleep problems, she was taking high blood pressure medicine and had frequent headaches. We referred Joan to a sleep lab for testing.

With all the electrodes, wires, and other apparatus that the sleep lab technicians had attached to her, Joan resembled a sleeping astronaut. At times, her chest was heaving, but she didn't seem to be moving air into her lungs. Her body jerked for up to a minute, sometimes longer, as if she were choking in her sleep. Then, suddenly, she let out an enormously loud, long, and violent snore. Then, silence. This happened over and over again during the test.

Since Joan had stopped breathing for ten seconds or more, more than five times each hour during the test, she was diagnosed with sleep apnea. Like her, some people with sleep apnea may stop breathing for as long as ninety seconds or more. The director of the sleep lab explained that Joan's brainwave tracings revealed that she spent little time in delta sleep—the very deep sleep that helps us feel well rested in the morning. When Joan wasn't breathing, the level of oxygen in her blood fell sharply. At times, the low oxygen levels caused her heart to beat somewhat irregularly. This is one major reason why approximately 50 percent of morbidly obese people with sleep apnea die in their sleep within eight years of developing this condition.

There are two main types of sleep apnea: *obstructive sleep apnea* and *central sleep apnea,* or a combination of the two. In central sleep apnea, the brain fails to properly pace one's breathing. In obstructive sleep apnea—the more common of the two—the airway becomes obstructed when the tongue loses its normal muscle tone during sleep and drops into the back of the throat. Morbidly obese people with sleep apnea usually have obstructive sleep apnea. This condition occurs in at least one in five morbidly obese people.

Sleep apnea is a very serious disorder, so it is vitally important that anyone with symptoms of this condition seeks medical attention. If indicated, most physicians will make a referral to a sleep lab for testing and diagnosis. Ninety percent of our weight-loss-surgery patients with obstructive sleep apnea were cured of this condition as a result of massive weight loss.

Urinary Stress Incontinence (Loss of Bladder Control)

When Dr. Cowan was a child, he witnessed an embarrassing moment in the life of a morbidly obese actress. She was doing a fine job acting her part, until she began coughing and a puddle of urine formed at her feet. The audience's peals of laughter greatly compounded her obvious distress. Dr. Cowan didn't understand the import, but he never forgot the event. It wasn't until many years later that he fully understood the problem.

The actress most likely suffered from urinary stress incontinence. This is a medical condition in which urine leaks out involuntarily during physical activities that increase the pressure within the abdomen, such as coughing, straining, laughing, lifting, and sneezing. This condition can occur in average-weight people as well as in obese individuals. However, in an obese person, intra-abdominal pressure is already one-half to two times greater than it is in a person of average weight due to excess body fat and larger muscle mass. This added pressure can overwhelm the proper function of the muscles that control the passage of urine. Therefore, an obese person's body is even less able to deal with the additional abdominal pressure caused by physical activities.

More than half of our female morbidly obese patients have this problem to a greater or lesser extent. (This condition can also affect men, but it occurs infrequently.) While there are operations meant to correct urinary stress incontinence, many of our obese patients who had these surgeries did not experience lasting improvement. After substantial weight loss, however, this problem cleared up in about 95 percent of our patients. In the remaining 5 percent, the problem seems to have causes unrelated to obesity, such as nerve or muscle damage associated with difficult childbirth.

Varicose Veins, Edema, and Leg Ulcers

Michael painfully lumbered into the exam room, tilting his body to one side and then to the other as he moved forward with the aid of a cane. Flesh bulged out over the tops of his unlaced triple-width shoes. The skin on the lower halves of his legs was spotted with large brown blotches, and the inner sides of his ankles were scarred. When Dr. Cowan pressed his finger into the skin on the front of Michael's leg, it made a dent about a half-inch deep that did not go away. Michael was obviously retaining massive amounts of water, but that wasn't the worst of his problems.

Michael's problems likely began with swelling in his legs due to excess water retention. As a result of the chronic swelling, the valves in the deep veins in his legs probably gave way so that the weight of the entire column of blood from his heart to his feet was so heavy that it caused his smaller veins to bulge and burst. This caused microscopic droplets of blood to form under, and in, his skin. As the red blood cells broke down, they turned brown, producing mottling. Michael had some heart failure, which added to the excess fluid in his lower limbs at this stage and caused him to breathe hard as he walked. The skin above his ankles was damaged by the excess pressure and formed ulcers, now healed into scars.

Many morbidly obese people have varicose veins—abnormally swollen or dilated veins—in the legs. Swelling of the ankles, feet, and legs are also common in people with varicose veins and can sometimes be disabling. At a later stage of this condition, the discoloration, fluid weeping from the skin, and ulcers of the legs, called *venous stasis ulcers,* may occur. After massive weight loss, edema usually resolves itself or, at least, becomes less pronounced. Varicose veins, however, do not resolve, may become more noticeable, and may require further medical attention.

Obesity and the Odds of Dying Prematurely

In a landmark study reported in the *Journal of the American Medical Association* in February 1980, Dr. Ernst J. Drenick and colleagues studied 200 morbidly obese men at UCLA over a seven-and-a-half-year period to determine the link between premature death and obesity. By the end of the study period, 25 percent of the subjects, many of whom were relatively young, had died.

Using these patients as a model, Drenick and colleagues calculated the chances of death in obese men versus the chances in their similar-height, average-weight counterparts. What they concluded is that a person between the ages of twenty-five and thirty-four has about a twelve times greater chance of dying prematurely than an average-weight person of the same age and sex. The researchers also concluded that an obese person has about a six to eight times greater chance of dying between the ages of thirty-five and forty-four than a non-obese counterpart. From forty-five years of age and greater, the risk is about three times greater. From the age of sixty years onward, weight does not appear to make a difference in death rate since average-weight people begin to die more frequently from heart disease, cancer, and other diseases; however, it's important to note that the vast majority of morbidly obese people die before reaching their sixtieth birthdays.

This tragic increase in the risk of death for the morbidly obese during their productive adult years is very significant—both personally and nationally. Obesity is undeniably an urgent health problem of vital importance. We're all entitled to a long, productive life, and weight-loss surgery can make that possible.

CONCLUSION

We hope this chapter has given you a better understanding of obesity and the health problems associated with it. You may be comforted to know that obesity is, in fact, classified as a disease. As you learned in this chapter, many of the health problems, or comorbidities, associated with this disease can be brought under control or even cured following massive weight loss.

As far as information goes, this is only the tip of the iceberg. There is much more you should know before deciding if weight-loss surgery is right for you. For starters, to seriously consider pursuing this surgery, you need to know if you might qualify for it. The next chapter will help you make this determination.

CHAPTER 2

$\mathscr{D}$O YOU QUALIFY FOR SURGERY?

Whether or not you qualify for weight-loss surgery may seem like a simple enough question on the surface. But when it comes to this body-altering surgery, the qualifications are not cut-and-dried. In the spring of 1991, a group of experts—including surgeons, gastroenterologists, psychiatrists, nutritionists, and other health-care professionals—gathered at the National Institutes of Health (NIH) Consensus Development Conference on Gastrointestinal Surgery for Severe Obesity. After reviewing the evidence presented at the conference, a consensus panel reached an agreement on the qualifications for weight-loss surgery. The guidelines set forth in their consensus statement have withstood the test of time and have remained the "gold standard" for determining who qualifies for weight-loss surgery. More recently, in May 2004, the American Society for Bariatric Surgery (ASBS) also held a consensus conference, and their guidelines complement the NIH's.

This chapter covers these official guidelines and also takes a look at the unofficial guidelines gathered from direct experience with thousands of patients. It also takes a look at the psychological and emotional qualifiers that play a role in making the decision to change one's life. Being familiar with these factors can help you determine if you are a good candidate for weight-loss surgery. Once you know if you qualify, you can then begin to make an informed decision about whether or not this surgery is right for you. This chapter closes with a brief discussion on the issue of health-insurance coverage. Whether or not your health-insurance provider will cover the cost of surgery is obviously another important factor to take into consideration.

QUALIFICATION GUIDELINES

The following sections take a close look at each of the qualifiers for weight-loss surgery, including body weight, evidence of previous weight-loss attempts, approval from a multidisciplinary team, and so on. Many of these factors are discussed in the NIH and ASBS guidelines. However, certain factors discussed here are properly left up to the surgeon's discretion.

Body Weight

The first consideration in determining if you qualify for weight-loss surgery is, of course, body weight—or more specifically, your body mass index (BMI). BMI is a measure of body fat based on height and weight. It is calculated by dividing your weight in kilograms by your height in meters squared. Your physician can tell you what your BMI is, or you can figure it out yourself. Here's how to do it with a calculator:

1. To find your weight in kilograms, divide your weight in pounds by 2.2.

   Your weight in kilograms: _____

2. To find your height in meters, multiply your height in inches by .0254.

   Your height in meters: _____

3. To find your height in meters squared, multiply your height in meters by itself.

   Your height in meters squared: _____

4. To find your BMI, divide your weight in kilograms by your height in meters squared.

   Your BMI: _____

A normal BMI is anywhere from 18 to 25. A BMI ranging from 26 to 29.9 is considered overweight, and a BMI of 30 and over is considered obese. If you have a BMI of 40 or more, you are classified as morbidly obese. This means that you are a definite candidate for surgery, but it is not a guarantee that a surgeon must or will accept you. Yes, it's an important first step toward qualifying for surgery, but there's more that a surgeon needs to know about you. To gather the necessary information, your surgeon will, among other things, review your medical history, have you undergo physical exams, consult with other health-care professionals and consider their evaluations, carefully consider lab results, and perform additional studies.

If your BMI is between 35 and 40, you may qualify for weight-loss surgery if you have a high-risk comorbidity, such as severe sleep apnea, type-2 diabetes, or physical problems that interfere with a normal lifestyle. These problems can include joint disease that cannot properly be treated due to the obesity and even less tangible problems such as being unable to get hired or hold a job. Another obesity-related problem that also interferes with a normal lifestyle is the inability to "get around." This can include difficulty traveling in cars, planes, trains, and buses, and even walking or standing at community events and other activities.

According to the NIH consensus guidelines, if your BMI is less than 35 you will not qualify for weight-loss surgery, regardless of any obesity-related conditions you might have. However, the ASBS's consensus statement, while otherwise agreeing with most of the NIH guidelines, suggests that, in the future, people with severe type-2 diabetes, sleep apnea, or similarly severe medical conditions, whose BMI is between 30 and 35, might benefit from this surgery. At first, this will need to be tested by research centers with strict guidelines for consideration for the surgery. If you are interested and think you might qualify, contact the American Society for Bariatric Surgery. (See the Resources section.)

Previous Weight-Loss Attempts

According to NIH and ASBS consensus guidelines, in order to qualify for surgery, you must show evidence of previous weight-loss attempts. Although research indicates that 98 percent of all morbidly obese people fail to lose weight and/or maintain the loss over the long term (three to five or more years) from diets, exercise, behavioral changes, or weight-loss medications (diet pills), a trial of these non-surgical weight-loss methods is still required by the guidelines.

With so much weight-loss advice and countless weight-loss diets on the market, it's no wonder that by the time a person visits a weight-loss surgeon's office for the first time (at the average age of thirty-six), her history of weight-loss attempts as recorded on a diet-report sheet usually goes back many years and includes all sorts of non-surgical weight-loss attempts, with temporary losses ranging from 0 to 100 pounds with each attempt.

Some health-insurance providers require patients to have years of documented physician-supervised weight-loss programs. This is unfair since there is no evidence that repeated weight-loss attempts do anything other than further delay a much-needed surgery. Nevertheless, if you are asked to fill out a diet-report sheet (or weight-loss-history report) at a surgeon's office, be sure to provide as detailed a list as possible of all your weight-loss attempts since this may influence your health-insurance provider's decision to approve the surgery. (There's more on health-insurance coverage later in the chapter and in Chapter 6.)

In our practice, if an obese person has not tried to lose weight with non-surgical methods, we will insist on a trial of diet therapy. However, practically all morbidly obese people have tried to lose weight in one way or another and have failed at least two or more times. Such a track record is usually acceptable to a surgeon.

Age

The NIH consensus guidelines do not include an upper limit on a person's age to qualify for surgery. However, both the NIH and ASBS panels found that too little evidence exists to support this surgery in those under age eighteen. As a result, weight-loss surgery is available to people under age eighteen only in certain weight-loss-surgery centers, assuming the person meets the same, or similar, qualifications as a qualifying adult.

Despite these panels' lack of recommendations for an upper-age limit, many weight-loss-surgery centers have cutoffs at age sixty and others accept very few patients over this age. Nevertheless, after very careful screening and evaluation, we have operated on people as old as age seventy-four and as young as age ten with good outcomes. The children's growth was not stunted as a result of the surgery, and they have done at least as well as our adult patients. Our elderly patients have done reasonably well following their weight-loss surgery, although they tend to lose somewhat less weight than their younger counterparts because their smaller muscle mass burns fewer calories.

In one case, an eighty-five-year-old morbidly obese woman, who very competently looked after her daughter following weight-loss surgery, asked coauthor Dr. Cowan if he would consider surgery in her case. She had practically no illnesses, so in Dr. Cowan's opinion, the risk of surgery outweighed the benefits. In another case, an obese seventy-five-year-old woman had significant arthritis but was in otherwise good health. She had not received good medical treatment for her arthritis nor had she ever tried to diet. In her case, we referred her to a nutritionist and an excellent arthritis specialist. If the specialist could not help her manage her crippling arthritis, we agreed to seriously consider her for weight-loss surgery. Although we knew that she could benefit from massive weight loss like many of our younger patients with similar problems, she was considerably older and, therefore, the risk of complications was higher. It was better for her to achieve her goal to walk without a walker, if possible, non-surgically.

Comorbidities

As mentioned earlier, in order for a person with a BMI between 35 and 39.9 to qualify for weight-loss surgery, she must have one or more comorbidities. Although the NIH consensus statement does not have such a requirement in cases of a BMI of 40 or higher, many health-insurance providers seem to prefer, or even require, two or more of these conditions to be present in order to approve coverage for the surgery. (See the list of medical conditions associated with obesity in Chapter 1.)

Don't forget that you may be unaware that you have such conditions. In the process of filling out the "tons" of paperwork required, be sure to provide detailed information about any health problems you may have had or have. This information coupled with the results of your tests will enable your surgeon to provide your health-insurance provider with a list of comorbidities that may satisfy their requirements.

Multidisciplinary Team Approval

The NIH consensus statement suggests that each potential weight-loss candidate be evaluated by a multidisciplinary team. This team includes a psychologist, psychiatrist, or social worker; a nutritionist; and medical/surgical specialists. Team members work together to determine if surgery is the best course of action. They will recommend against this route if a person is, in their professional opinions, clearly not a candidate or if she would benefit from some specialized treatment before having the surgery.

Here's an example: Sandra was not a good surgical candidate because our team psychologist determined that she was significantly depressed. Depression, or a history of depression, would not necessarily prevent you from having weight-loss surgery; in fact, a large percentage of our patients do have some degree of depression. However, Sandra's depression was serious, and she needed to receive treatment to bring it under control. Otherwise, she was at risk of becoming even more depressed as a result of the changes that occur in brain chemistry brought on by massive weight loss. When Sandra's psychiatrist reported that she was stable for three months with treatment, our multidisciplinary team cleared her for surgery. Sandra agreed to continue therapy and to remain on antidepressants until at least three months after her weight loss had leveled off. The surgery went just fine, and she continued to take the antidepressants as she had agreed. Now, years later, she has lost most of her excess weight and no longer takes medication. She looks and feels very good, and there's no hint of her previous depression.

If a person does not receive treatment for significant depression before surgery, she may later wind up with a major crisis. (There's more on the risk of depression following weight-loss surgery in Chapter 8.)

Informed Consent

The NIH and ASBS consensus statements also indicate that, in order to be accepted for surgery, a person must be well informed. This means that a surgical candidate must be provided with information that can be reasonably understood and that adequately explains the proposed surgery, other surgical and non-surgical options, the risks and complications associated with this and other surgery, and the expected benefits.

In addition to receiving this information, you should be given the opportunity to have all your questions answered to your satisfaction by the surgeon. Such questions may include how many weight-loss surgeries the

---

Do You Have Your Family's Support?

When you're considering having weight-loss surgery, it's ideal to have your family's support. If you have the surgery, you will surely need their assistance down the road. You will be going through major changes—both emotional and physical—and it will be impossible to hide this from them.

Although there are no official guidelines regarding a support system, this is a very significant consideration. In our practice, we prefer to be assured that, at the very least, a person's spouse or significant other supports her decision to have the surgery. Fortunately, this is usually the case.

It's best to be upfront with your family members and friends so that they can be prepared for the changes that will take place. Share with them any literature you read on the topic, including this book. They may find Part Four particularly helpful since it was written especially for them. Also see Chapter 4 for some helpful advice for telling those closest to you about your possible decision to have the surgery.

potential surgeon has performed and what the results were. Be sure to ask about anything that comes to mind. Since you may be a little nervous during your office visit with the surgeon, make a list of all your questions before the office visit so that you cover everything you can while you have the chance to do so. (See Chapter 4 for a helpful questionnaire you may want to use.)

Having all the details helps you understand that there is nothing magical about this surgery. To be a good candidate for weight-loss surgery, you must be completely realistic about what you are facing in the way of surgery and its lifelong effects, both positive and negative. Then, you must realistically weigh the risks of serious problems against the potential benefits.

Willingness to Carry Out Instructions

In order to be considered for surgery, you must be willing and able to carry out your surgeon's instructions—not only around the time of surgery but for the remainder of your life. This includes faithfully returning to the surgeon's office for follow-up appointments as instructed and remaining under watchful medical care for life.

Precautions Against Pregnancy

Women who are in their reproductive years should agree to take every precaution to avoid becoming pregnant for eighteen months to two years following weight-loss surgery. While you may wish to get started on a family or add to your family right away, your body will be in no condition to deal with the stress of pregnancy. If you neglect this instruction and become pregnant, the developing fetus will drain your body of some much-needed nutrition during your weight loss. Not only could this harm you, but it could also harm your baby, particularly if you become malnourished.

Dozens of our patients have successfully had children, but the risks are very real. If you do become pregnant, you must be closely monitored, particularly to make sure no nutritional deficiencies occur that could harm you or your unborn child. (See the inset "Wait to Become Pregnant" on page 160 in Chapter 9 for more information.)

No Excessive Risk

According to the NIH consensus statement, candidates for weight-loss surgery must be able to tolerate the surgery "without excessive risk." As individual surgeons gain more experience performing these operations, they can perform the surgery without excessive risk on people with higher BMIs who are somewhat more ill. In fact, surgeons usually make their own judgments concerning who they think is able to tolerate the surgery. If a person is too heavy, too ill, or displays uncooperative behavior, a surgeon may have reservations about accepting her for the procedure due to the excessive risk involved. In some cases, a potential candidate will be asked to lose some weight, sometimes a large amount, to achieve some level of health to be reconsidered for surgery. A person who cannot or refuses to cooperate with the surgeon and staff will not be favorably considered for surgery, since her noncompliance would create an excessive risk.

Obese people with severe medical problems who are unlikely to tolerate surgery or a major surgery-related complication will be turned away. A person with congestive heart failure, for instance, would not qualify. In such a case, the person's heart is pumping only enough blood to keep her alive and, therefore, could not tolerate the additional stress of anesthesia and surgery. Likewise, a person with moderate to severe pulmonary hypertension, abnormally high pressure in the blood vessels to the lungs, is highly unlikely to fare well under anesthesia and after the surgery. Nevertheless, we have performed surgery on people with relatively mild forms of pulmonary hypertension and, together with the assistance of a lung specialist, have been able to get good results after surgery.

Also, people with severe liver disease may not fare well following weight-loss surgery. So, if it is known that severe liver disease is present, most surgeons will conclude that the risk is too great. Unfortunately, in some cases, liver disease is discovered only after the surgery has begun. Whether or not to proceed with the surgery at that point is a matter of the surgeon's judgment.

People with a history of blood clots (deep venous thrombosis) or clots that travel to the lungs (pulmonary emboli) usually require special handling before we consider them for surgery. Likewise, people with thyroid disease or diabetes also require special consideration. These disorders need to be under adequate control before surgery is considered. If these disorders are not controlled, they can increase the risks of complications, and fall under the category of "excessive risk."

No Substance Abuse

Substance abuse and weight-loss surgery are a potentially lethal combination. Therefore, alcoholics and illicit drug users will not be considered for weight-loss surgery. In our practice, we have refused any person who cannot demonstrate at least six months of complete sobriety prior to surgery.

AIDS-Free

An obese person with AIDS will likely experience malnutrition due to the disease and will inevitably lose weight. Therefore, to perform weight-loss surgery on such a person is highly questionable. There's a good possibility that the surgery would have to be reversed due to malnourishment. However, a newer type of surgery that can be "reversed" non-surgically might be acceptable in certain carefully selected cases. (See page 40 in Chapter 3 for a discussion on adjustable gastric banding.)

PSYCHOLOGICAL AND EMOTIONAL QUALIFIERS

The guidelines for weight-loss surgery discussed above are, of course, essential in determining who qualifies for surgery. However, simply being a good candidate for weight-loss surgery doesn't mean you will choose to have surgery. The discussions to follow and, most important, the patients' stories included in these sections and elsewhere in the book can help you decide if weight-loss surgery is right for you. We hear stories like theirs—and yours—practically every day in our office. The stories are painful, courageous, and compelling. All of the patients mentioned throughout this book have successfully completed weight-loss surgery. They would all tell you that their decision was a serious and thoughtful one, as yours should be. While each person is unique, all of our patients shared one thing in common: morbid obesity controlled every area of their lives and they were not willing to continue to live that way. Weight-loss surgery provided them with new hope and a chance to fulfill their dreams. Perhaps you will decide that it can do the same for you.

An Awareness of an Increased Risk of Imminent Death

Although you may be well aware of the many health-related side effects of your obesity, it is often possible to pretend that they don't exist—sometimes for a very long time. After a while, denial can become an almost normal part of getting through your daily life. Then, one day, you visit your doctor—perhaps just for a routine visit—and like our patient Frank, you hear the words, "If you do not lose weight, you will die." This is the first unofficial qualifier—the complete and utter realization that your health and weight have become life threatening. Although you may have been told at some point in the past that morbid obesity can decrease your life expectancy by fifteen years, that probably felt so far away—some distant point in the future. But this is immediate: something must be done or you will not survive.

The Desire for a Better Quality of Life

In general, people who decide to have weight-loss surgery have experienced a compromised quality of life. Their activities and options have been severely limited by their weight. Some people describe feeling like they are living in an older person's body even though they are only middle-aged. Many of our morbidly obese patients experience constant pain and, even more significantly, live in constant fear—a fear not only of dying but also of living. Their obesity affects the way they feel every day.

Cathy, a talented writer and single mother, describes her concerns regarding quality-of-life issues this way: "I'm thirty-four years old and weigh 280 pounds—that's more than twice my ideal body weight. My BMI is 50. My head hurts, my jaw hurts, and my shoulders, knees, and back hurt. I'll probably have diabetes by the time I'm forty. For now, my blood pressure is in the normal range, but what will the next few years bring? I don't want to be reliant on insulin and an oxygen tank. I want to be able to walk up the street or climb a flight of stairs without becoming short of breath. Despite my serious efforts, I keep gaining more weight. With more weight comes more problems. I want to enjoy my life. I want to be healthy." Another patient, Wendy, describes her quality-of-life issues this way: "The bigger I get, the smaller my options become."

Even the simplest things that most people take for granted are monumental tasks for people who are morbidly obese. They can barely move, breathe, climb steps, bend over to tie their shoes, or even complete some of the most basic tasks of hygiene. It's impossible for them to buy clothes in a regular clothing store, and average-size jewelry often does not fit their necks or wrists. Restaurants, theaters, and movies are not chosen for the quality of the food or entertainment but for the width of the seating. Walking through turnstiles and down aisles can become complex maneuvers. Even simply walking to the mailbox can become a subject for contemplation.

Quality of life has so many facets, including numerous sexual and physical limitations—so many, in fact, that it's impossible to mention them all. But you probably already know all about them and how these limitations can contribute to a diminished quality of life. Considering weight-loss surgery for its potential to improve your quality of life is yet another qualifier.

The Realization That Diets Just Don't Work

In some areas, weight-loss-surgery candidates must show evidence of two medically supervised weight-loss attempts and/or provide a history of unsupervised weight-loss attempts in order to qualify for surgery. Many of our patients claim this is the easiest part of the process since they've been on diets for most of their lives. Many of these diets were supervised by weight-loss centers, doctors' offices, clinics, and in-patient hospital programs, and may have also included supervised exercise programs. And, unfortunately, most of these diets failed. In fact, popular and medical literature is rampant with articles on why diets don't work.

Wendy says, "Over the past twenty-one years, I've lost and gained about 550 pounds. Between exercise programs, gym memberships, gimmicks, exercise equipment, and fees for diet plans like Jenny Craig and Weight Watchers, I've probably spent over $10,000, and guess what, I'm heavier than ever!" Another patient, Mike, says, "My weight has been a problem since age five. I've been fighting the battle for fifty years, winning only temporary victories. I have been on Weight Watchers, the rice diet, high-protein/low-carb diets, amphetamines, thyroid pills, Prozac, liquid protein, fasts, acupuncture, Overeaters Anonymous, and a series of other therapies that have faded from my weary memory. I'm throwing in the towel!"

We hear stories like Wendy's and Mike's every day. So many obese people are tired of hearing their well-meaning friends and family members, and, at times, even their physicians saying, "If only you would go on a diet. . . ." Most of our patients have gone on virtually every known diet. On the whole, they've been diligent and have worked hard, and, in some cases, have lost weight, perhaps a substantial amount. However, although they successfully lost weight, they eventually gained it back with perhaps more than they lost. At some point, it becomes crystal clear that weight-loss diets just don't work for the morbidly obese over the long term, and this becomes another qualifier for surgery.

Recognizing the Genetic Role in Obesity

In the past, people were generally not accepting of the notion that obesity is a genetic problem. With the tremendous advances in knowledge that are occurring every day in the field of obesity, we are finding out that obesity clearly has a strong genetic component. Cathy's story clearly illustrates the point: She had been adopted into a family of non-obese people who were generally healthy. Despite their average weight, she became obese and was teased about it all throughout her childhood. When she reached adulthood, she went in search of her birth family. "I couldn't believe it!" said Cathy. "Everyone in my birth family was obese! Nobody seemed to care about my

size, and they loved me for me! Most of all, I'd finally found the answer to
the question that had been plaguing me since I was twelve, 'why me?' "

When obese people learn that there really is a genetic component and
that their obesity may not be their fault, their longstanding feelings of
immobility, helplessness, shame, and guilt are lifted, thereby empowering
them. They begin to realize that they deserve a better life, and start to think
that weight-loss surgery may be the answer to counteract this genetic
component.

Tired of Being the Victim of Weight Prejudice

If you are morbidly obese, you probably don't have to be told how cruel
and abusive people with a weight prejudice can be. The profound emotional fallout of ongoing weight prejudice—in the family, from the community, and on the job—can severely compromise and limit all aspects of a
morbidly obese person's life. You've probably heard things like: "You have
such a pretty face; if only you'd lose some weight." Or "Why don't you just
control yourself and get up from the table!" Remarks like these probably
want to make you scream. Unfortunately, the bottom line is, wherever you
go and whatever you do, if you are morbidly obese, the first thing many
people will notice about you is your weight—and, in some cases, that's all
they will see. Wendy says, "What I dream about is being in a room where
everyone sees me as more than that 'fat girl in the corner.' I want them to
see a kind person with a radiant smile and a big heart." Does Wendy's
dream sound familiar? It sounds so simple on the surface, but the dream is
almost impossible to attain if people cannot see past the weight and into the
real person inside.

In some cases, weight prejudice may come from the most innocent
sources. For example, Mike was a well-respected professor who traveled
around the world. At 340 pounds, he was a rarity in China and was constantly asked questions not about life in the United States but about his
weight. And Tim, another patient, remembers how it felt when small children pointed at him and said, "Look at that fat man!" Now, 120 pounds
lighter, Tim gladly reports that he is now virtually invisible in public! Tina,
meanwhile, experienced less-than-innocent weight prejudice. She says, "At
two hundred pounds overweight, I felt like people were overwhelmed by
my presence—like I was taking up their space. I felt as visible as a billboard
and couldn't get through a day without experiencing anger and hatred. I
was reminded over and over that I repulsed, embarrassed, and humiliated
people just by being around. I often felt like I was perceived as a thing, not

a person—pointed out, made fun of, criticized, ignored, or passed over. The simplest tasks became torture when other people were around, and I became great at ignoring verbal attacks, hostility, and aggression in private and in public. People say get over it, that's the way life is, take it with a grain of salt. I feel differently. Weight prejudice is like a paper cut, you can ignore it, but hundreds of paper cuts add up to a life-threatening wound." In making the serious decision about whether weight-loss surgery is for you, consider Tina's statement—have your paper cuts added up to a life-threatening wound?

There's a good chance you recognized yourself in the above sections and understand the psychological and emotional qualifiers only too well. When making your decision, keep in mind that weight-loss surgery can help you attain life-long health and perhaps lasting happiness. Meanwhile, to close this chapter, let's take a look at the issue of health insurance, an important consideration.

QUALIFYING FOR HEALTH-INSURANCE COVERAGE

Most people cannot cover the cost of weight-loss surgery on their own—the average cost is $25,000, but it can range from $15,000 to $50,000. And that's assuming there are no complications. Major complications resulting from the surgery could add hundreds of thousands of dollars to the hospital bill.

It seems only reasonable that when a health-insurance provider enters into a contract with you to cover your health care that it should be obligated to pay for whatever it takes to keep or make you healthy. In an ideal world, when a weight-loss surgeon informs your insurance carrier that surgery is medically necessary for your health, the insurance company would approve the surgery. Unfortunately, this is not always what happens. Fortunately, there are steps you can take to increase the chances that you will receive approval.

For starters, if you've made the decision that surgery is right for you, make an appointment to see your primary-care physician (PCP). Your PCP should be familiar with your medical history and may even be aware of your failed attempts to lose weight. Discuss your decision with your PCP and ask her for a referral to the weight-loss surgeon you've selected. With your PCP's referral and support, your insurance provider is more likely to cover the surgeon's initial consultation and the cost of the surgery.

If your PCP does not agree that weight-loss surgery is right for you and will not give you a referral, find another PCP for a second opinion. If you already have a weight-loss surgeon in mind, contact the surgeon's office and ask for a list of PCPs in your area who have referred patients to that surgeon. There's a chance you may have to contact several PCPs who are approved by your health-insurance company to find one who can help you. Call each office and ask the nurse whether or not the doctor refers patients for weight-loss surgery. When you find one that does, make an appointment.

Also, gather letters in support of the surgery from other physicians who have treated you for obesity-related conditions, such as urinary stress incontinence, back pain, knee problems, or sleep apnea. Such letters can help sway the decision in your favor. Before these letters are submitted to your health-insurance provider, be sure to review them carefully to make sure they do, in fact, support your surgery. Provide your weight-loss surgeon with copies of these letters so she can use them to support your need for surgery when contacting your health-insurance company.

The majority of health-insurance providers will cover weight-loss surgery if the requirements are met. However, some insurance companies have "disqualifiers" or lists of procedures they will not cover, and, unfortunately, weight-loss surgery may be one of them. If you come up against an insurance roadblock, your surgeon may be able to try different approaches to get approval that have worked for other people. For instance, if a policy states that it does not cover *obesity* but fails to mention *morbid obesity* and you are morbidly obese, there may be some room to work with the insurer in order to obtain coverage. In other cases, a policy may state that *obesity treatment* is not covered but does not specifically state that *obesity surgery* is not covered. In such cases, the surgery may be covered.

Sometimes, health-insurance providers have their own rules regarding the qualifications for surgery. For instance, some may actually require that you be *twice* your ideal body weight or, in at least one case we know of, *two and a half times* your ideal body weight. This far exceeds the NIH guidelines and strikes many people and health-care professionals as unfair. Moreover, some health-insurance providers may require that patients have up to a five-year history of consecutive, unsuccessful weight-loss treatments, all documented in writing. Fortunately, many insurance companies have dropped this outrageous requirement but, in some cases, have substituted other requirements that seem just as unreasonable.

Keep in mind that, if your insurance company initially denies coverage for the surgery, you can appeal the decision. Many of our patients have won their appeals.

People who have the resources to pay for weight-loss surgery out of pocket are very fortunate. However, even if you are one of these people, you should discuss your coverage with your insurance representative. In the case of complications, you could be facing a huge hospital bill that you did not plan for. A few hospitals that have weight-loss surgery programs will agree to put a cap on the maximum amount a self-paying patient must pay for the surgery, regardless of possible excessive costs due to complications. If this applies to you, consider insisting on such an arrangement with the hospital prior to your surgery.

If you are finding it very difficult to get coverage, find out how other people in your situation successfully obtained coverage. Support groups and Internet groups, especially those affiliated with the surgeon you have chosen, should be able to provide you will helpful information about how to effectively navigate the insurance maze. (For more information on insurance coverage, see Chapter 6.)

CONCLUSION

We hope this chapter has addressed all of your questions concerning your qualifications for weight-loss surgery. You should now have some idea if a surgeon will accept you for surgery and if your health-insurance provider will cover it. Also, you probably recognized yourself in the section on emotional and psychological qualifiers; chances are you've come to those very same realizations even before you picked up this book. When deciding if the surgery is right for you, these are all important factors to take into consideration. Still, you probably need more questions answered before making your final decision—for instance, what type of surgery options will be available to you and what exactly do they entail? The next chapter will provide you with some important information.

CHAPTER 3

*W*HICH OPTION IS RIGHT FOR YOU?

I f you are obese or morbidly obese, you know how rare it is to feel full after eating. In fact, you may never have felt this way. This lack of feeling full is probably one of the main reasons you keep gaining weight despite dieting efforts, behavior-modification courses, regular exercise, and weight-loss medications. Weight-loss surgery enables you to feel full after eating by surgically reducing the size of your stomach.

Certain types of weight-loss surgery involve separating a portion of the uppermost part of the stomach from the lower part of the stomach. This separate upper part becomes what is called the *stomach pouch* or *gastric pouch.* Following most types of weight-loss surgery, it usually takes only 1–3 ounces of food to fill the pouch. When the pouch walls are stretched by this little amount of food, a strong message to stop eating is sent to the brain. These messages enable a person who has undergone weight-loss surgery to feel full, often for the first time in his life. This person is now in control of eating and is satisfied with far less food than before the surgery. As a result of stomach reduction—sometimes together with surgery on the small intestines—the person loses weight. Although it is unclear exactly how the "I'm full" messages get through, we do not need to understand the exact details to know that stomach reduction works for almost anyone who undergoes it. In time, research will tell us more.

This chapter takes a look at surgical approaches (laparoscopic and open methods) and your surgery options (restrictive bariatric surgery and malabsorptive bariatric surgery, and their variations). While there are many different types of surgery, they all have the same ultimate goals: to help you lose weight and regain your health and well-being.

SURGICAL APPROACHES TO WEIGHT-LOSS SURGERY

There are two surgical approaches to performing all of the different types of weight-loss, or bariatric, surgery: open or laparoscopic. As you'll learn in the sections to follow, each has its advantages and disadvantages. To date, the overall percentage of complications that can occur in the first thirty days after either surgical approach is about equal in the hands of highly experienced surgeons. However, laparoscopic bariatric surgery seems to be overtaking the open approach as the more popular choice. Nevertheless, both types of surgery require an extended recovery time—at least two to four weeks following laparoscopic bariatric surgery and six weeks following open bariatric surgery.

Open Approach

Open bariatric surgery has been around for more than fifty years and is still performed today. In this surgical approach, an incision is usually made from the lower end of the breastbone to the area above, or beside, the bellybutton, technically referred to as the *umbilicus.* The open approach gives the surgeon a good view and feel of the patient's abdominal organs during the procedure. In about 10 to 30 percent of patients, a ventral hernia (see page 165) may develop in the opening postsurgically. An operation to correct this complication is usually necessary.

Following open weight-loss surgery, a person will usually experience some pain at the site of the surgical incision, which is controlled with pain medicine given by vein (intravenously), by injections in the arm or buttock muscle or, later, by mouth. Except in unusual cases, most people are discharged from the hospital within two to five days, with their pain, if any, acceptably controlled with medication.

Laparoscopic Approach

In laparoscopic bariatric surgery, which has been more generally available for the past ten years or so, the surgeon works with a fiber-optic video camera and other specialized instruments through five to eight one-inch or so openings in the front of the abdomen called *ports,* instead of the larger, open-approach incision. These smaller incisions usually cause less discomfort than the larger incision and most often result in a shorter recovery time. Furthermore, there is less stress to the body overall with this type of surgery.

This approach is not without complications, however. The bowel, bladder, blood vessels, or a nerve can be damaged during the insertion of some of the surgical equipment. In this case and for other technical reasons, such as a very large liver obscuring the stomach, a surgeon may have to switch over to the open method during the surgery. The more experience a surgeon has, the less frequently this should be necessary.

Laparoscopic surgery is usually associated with costs that amount to $2,000 to $3,000 more than open surgery. This is due to the special equipment required—for example additional stapler cartridges and other disposable equipment. For this reason, among others, health-insurance providers in certain states have been reluctant to approve the laparoscopic approach; however, this reluctance appears to be lessening.

RESTRICTIVE BARIATRIC SURGERY

In restrictive bariatric surgery—the first of the two surgical options—the surgeon fashions a small pouch from the upper part of the stomach and does not operate upon the intestines. The pouch and narrowed pouch outlet work by physically *restricting* the amount of food that can be eaten at any one time. This type of surgery usually results in weight loss of anywhere from one-third to somewhat more than one-half of the patient's excess weight. Along with the weight loss, comorbidities often improve or disappear.

Restrictive bariatric surgery is not for everyone, however. The main problem with this type of surgery is that it drastically limits the amount of food and liquids a person can consume at any one time. This can result in nausea and vomiting if more food is swallowed than can fit in the pouch before it empties. However, a good degree of restriction is necessary in restrictive bariatric surgery in order to produce sufficient weight loss by means of altering only the stomach. On the other hand, malabsorptive bariatric surgeries (discussed on page 42) do not require as much stomach restriction since they also produce weight loss by reducing the amount of food the intestines can absorb. Therefore, food intake is not as limited, and the nausea and vomiting associated with restrictive surgery is less of a problem.

People who have restrictive weight-loss surgery must eat very small amounts of food at each meal; they must eat slowly and chew their food thoroughly until it is liquefied. Moreover, they must eat frequently to adequately nourish themselves. Some people find this intolerable. Others eat more food than they should at one sitting and become ill. Others complain that it's embarrassing to eat so little in front of others. However, many people who have undergone restrictive bariatric surgery are quite proud of their newfound "control" over food and revel in the feeling of fullness and the weight loss that comes with it.

Typically, a person chooses restrictive bariatric surgery over malabsorptive bariatric surgery because he wants a relatively simpler, less-risky option and is willing to do whatever must be done after surgery, including eating more slowly, chewing more thoroughly, and "obeying" the signals that it's time to stop eating sooner than with a malabsorptive procedure. Some may choose this type of surgery because they want to avoid the side effects of the more complex surgeries discussed later in this chapter—such as unexpected urgent bowl movements and "dumping syndrome," also called *rapid gastric emptying*—when food and/or liquid passes too quickly into the rectum or small intestines (see page 48).

Today, the two main types of restrictive bariatric surgery are gastroplasty and adjustable gastric banding. These are discussed below.

Gastroplasty

From the 1980s through the mid-1990s, gastroplasty was by far the most frequently performed bariatric surgery procedure. This was due in part to the enormous influence of its inventor, Dr. Edward E. Mason of the University of Iowa. Today, gastroplasty is performed in fewer than 10 percent of cases.

Dr. Mason coined the term *gastroplasty* from the prefix *gastro,* which means "stomach" and the suffix *plasty,* which means "molding or forming surgically." In this procedure, the surgeon "reshapes" the upper part of the stomach into a two-or-so-inch-long tube using surgical staples. (Food and liquid will pass along this tube and then move through its narrowed exit, called the *stoma,* into the rest of the stomach.) Next, to set this narrowing at the surgeon's chosen diameter, a plastic band or ring is placed completely around the pouch stoma. Its purpose is to keep the opening of the pouch stoma—which is about as small as the end digit of an average-sized pinky finger—from becoming wider than intended. Even a few millimeters of extra stomal enlargement can result in long-term weight-loss failure.

Dr. Mason learned early on that, if some restriction such as a band were not placed around the pouch, his patients' eating habits would gradually cause the pouch to enlarge so much that it was no longer restricting food from reaching the main part of the stomach. Then, with food freely entering the stomach once again, these patients stopped losing weight and started to regain it.

Vertical banded gastroplasty (VBG) and, its variant, Silastic ring gastroplasty (SRG), are the two main types of gastroplasty. These surgeries are generally referred to as *stomach stapling.* This term is only correctly used when describing surgeries in which only the stomach itself is stapled.

Take a look at Figure 3.1 below. This figure illustrates a VBG. Notice the small hole in the stomach. The surgeon makes a round hole through both stomach walls with a circular cutter-stapler about an inch to the left of the lesser (shorter) curve of the stomach. He then wraps a rectangular strip of plastic mesh through the hole and around the shorter (lesser) curve of the stomach to form a small, non-stretchable, outlet stoma. Surgeons may use other types of rings and bands to reinforce the pouch stoma. These include Teflon, Goretex, Silastic rubber (hence *Silastic ring gastroplasty,* or *SRG*), and fibrous connective tissue taken from the front of the abdominal wall during surgery.

In VBG, the vertically stapled stomach walls may sometimes pull apart from each other, which occurs in 1 to 8 percent of cases each year. This separation can occur months, or even years, after surgery. When this happens, food is no longer restricted when it passes through the pouch into the lower stomach. As a result, the person no longer "feels full" and will regain much, if not all, of the lost weight. In an effort to prevent this from happening, many surgeons completely cut through the stomach between the vertical staple lines. By doing this, the staples seal off either side of the now almost completely separated stomach. When the vertical edges (or *stumps,* as they

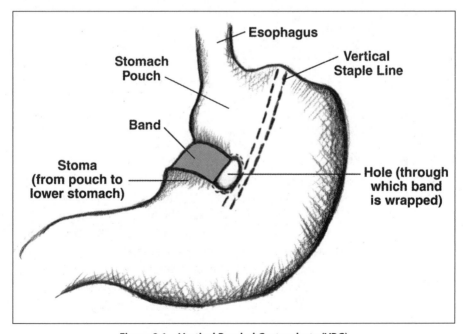

Figure 3.1. Vertical Banded Gastroplasty (VBG)

Surgical Staplers—A Marvelous Invention But Not Without Risks

The surgical stapler, which is used in many types of surgeries, is a very useful medical device that allows for quicker operating time during complex procedures. The high-quality staples used are made of rust-proof surgical steel. Some people fear that these staples will set off metal detectors, but there is no cause for concern. The staples used for the VBG and the SRG are very small, not magnetic, and lie deep within the abdomen; they cannot set off these types of alarms.

Like anything else, surgical stapling can have its downside. In about a 0.5 to 8 percent of cases, the staples do not work as expected, and, as a result, the stomach or the intestine leaks its contents into the abdominal cavity or bleeding occurs. A surgeon checks for and repairs leaks and bleeding during surgery and in the few days following surgery. Drains may be placed during the operation or later to control leakage. In some cases of leaks or bleeding, emergency surgery may be necessary. Although rare, this complication can be quite serious and life threatening. It will, at the very least, lengthen the hospital stay.

are called) heal, the dense scarring on each stump keeps the walls permanently sealed. In very rare cases, however, these two stomach stumps can "rechannel" across the staple lines to rejoin the pouch with the lower stomach, thereby ruining the surgery's purpose.

Gastric Banding

In the other main type of restrictive bariatric surgery, gastric banding, a band is wrapped around the upper part of the stomach to form a small pouch. This is done without using a surgical stapler or cutting into the stomach walls. Non-adjustable, or fixed, stomach bands have been around for more than twenty-five years, and some weight-loss surgery centers still use them. However, *adjustable* gastric bands (AGBs) have become the preferred type of band. The majority of bariatric surgeries performed outside of the United States are AGBs; the bands are manufactured by at least five different companies. Only one company, INAMED, currently has a band, called the *Lap-Band*, that is approved by the U.S. Food and Drug Administration (FDA). In time, additional bands will likely receive FDA approval for use in this country.

In adjustable gastric banding, an inflatable plastic band is wrapped around the upper stomach without any stapling or cutting of the stomach. The band comes with a thin tube that connects it to a small metal cylinder called a *port* that is placed deep into the fat and skin of the upper abdomen. Depending upon each surgeon's usual practice, fluid is injected through the patient's skin and into the port at various times. This causes a balloon inside the band to inflate with the fluid. As more fluid is injected into the port, the balloon presses inward on the pouch stoma causing it to get smaller and more restrictive. (Some surgeons partially inflate the balloon during surgery, but others may wait a month or more after surgery.) Each surgeon develops a schedule of band inflation that appears to work best for his patients. Some have rigid, calendar-marked schedules that involve injecting a fixed amount of fluid into the band (through the port under the skin) at intervals of so many weeks or months. Other surgeons "tailor" the fluid injections; that is, they inject (and sometimes remove) varying amounts of fluid that, in their judgment, best manage their patients' weight-loss needs. Some surgeons find x-ray equipment helpful to help make their adjustments.

The advantage of adjustability is that fluid can be removed from the balloon if a problem, such as excessive nausea or vomiting, arises. Also, more fluid can be added to the balloon to make the pouch stoma smaller if food intake needs to be further restricted for additional weight loss.

People choose the AGB usually because they want a relatively low-risk procedure that will improve or eliminate many of their comorbidities—even though the average person who undergoes this type of surgery only loses about one-half, or slightly less, of his excess body weight. Although results vary from center to center, this is usually somewhat less than the weight loss reported for the VBG or SRG. With these surgeries, weight loss occurs in the first nine to eighteen months. With AGB, however, weight loss can continue for up to three years depending upon the inflation schedule for the band and the individual's response to the increasing restriction due to the inflation.

People also choose AGB because they like the fact that the band can be partially or completely deflated to allow them to consume more food with fewer problems during periods of need, such as with excessive nausea and vomiting related to pregnancy or otherwise. Also, since AGB does not involve stapling or cutting the stomach, the surgery can be relatively simply reversed by band removal.

Some surgeons recommend AGBs for people who, for example, have chronic anemia (a condition in which the blood is deficient in red blood cells, in hemoglobin, or in total volume) or an intestinal disorder such as Crohn's disease, or who refuse blood or blood products under any circumstance, such as Jehovah's Witnesses. Other surgeons recommend the AGB because this is the only weight-loss procedure they perform; in this case, you may need to "shop around" to seek the advice of surgeons who perform other, not purely restrictive, procedures before deciding what is best for you.

Band displacement, also called *band migration,* is a complication that occurs when part of the stomach wall "moves," or migrates, inside the circle of the band. This usually causes the pouch to empty more slowly than usual, since the migration of the stomach wall has partially, or completely, obstructed the pouch stoma. Another type of band migration causes the band to become tilted, thereby kinking the pouch stoma and preventing the pouch from emptying into the rest of the stomach. Band migration can occur in about 5 percent of cases, although the rate varies among surgeons. If this complication occurs, additional surgery may be necessary to place the migrated band back into its proper position.

In less than 1 percent of cases, a band may wear a hole through the stomach wall and erode into the inside of the stomach itself. The eroded band can sometimes be removed with the use of a scope passed through the mouth. Sometimes surgery is necessary to remove the eroded band. Other complications can occur, as well. For instance, the small band tubing may become infected, leak, or develop a bad connection with its port and not keep the band properly inflated. Surgery to repair this problem can often take place just under the skin and fat layer on the abdominal wall, but reoperation inside the abdominal cavity may be necessary. In these instances, the procedure is relatively straightforward and low risk.

In a few cases, a person who has had this procedure will develop a markedly enlarged esophagus due to the presence of the band. Why this condition occurs in some people and not in others is unclear. It has been reported more frequently in the United States than in Europe or elsewhere. It usually responds to band deflation or removal. Depending upon the success of the surgery to start with, if reoperation becomes necessary, some people may ask to be "converted" to another type of surgery associated with greater amounts of weight loss.

MALABSORPTIVE BARIATRIC SURGERY

While restrictive bariatric surgery only limits the intake of food, malabsorptive bariatric surgery—the second of the two surgical options—also limits the body's absorption of food by altering the digestive process. This new digestive hook-up appears to result in additional, or strengthened,

"I'm full" messages to the brain. With this type of surgery, some food intake is lost in bowel movements and is not absorbed by the body; hence, the term *malabsorption*. Because of this added effect, malabsorptive surgery tends to result in greater weight loss than restrictive surgery. For example, people who undergo regular gastric bypass surgery (see below) tend to lose an average of 10 to 15 percent more excess weight than people who undergo restrictive procedures.

Malabsorptive procedures do have greater risks associated with them, however. Some people are willing to take this risk to achieve greater weight loss. Once the decision to have this type of surgery is made, the next decision involves how much malabsorption is enough. To better understand this choice and related issues, let's first look at the basic and mildest type of malabsorptive bariatric surgery—regular gastric bypass surgery. Then we'll look at the more involved procedures.

Regular Gastric Bypass (GBP) Surgery (or Roux-en-Y Gastric Bypass)

In regular gastric bypass surgery, also called *Roux-en-Y gastric bypass*, the surgeon forms a small stomach pouch similar to the pouch formed in restrictive bariatric surgery. However, in this surgery, the stomach pouch is completely separated from the bottom part of the stomach by stapling and, most frequently, by completely dividing the stomach from itself between the rows of staples (see Figure 3.2 on page 44). Any food or liquid swallowed will "bypass" this now-separated, lower stomach. The "food stomach" is the pouch through which food and liquids will pass after they are eaten. The "bypassed stomach" will remain empty except for the acid and digestive juices that it will continue to produce.

Each of these two stomachs—the "food stomach" (the pouch) and the "bypassed stomach" (the digestive-juice stomach)—empty into two different limbs of the small intestine formed by the surgeon. The food stomach empties into a 2- to 5-foot-long food limb, and the bypassed stomach empties into the uppermost part of the small intestine called the *duodenum*, as it did before the surgery.

Another way to look at this surgery is to envision the capital letter "Y" in the term *Roux-en-Y*. In the original nineteenth-century procedure performed for other reasons, the Swiss surgeon Dr. Cesar Roux (1857–1934) fashioned the shape of a capital letter "Y" out of the small intestines. That is, one of the two slanted limbs at the top of the "Y" is attached to the small pouch through which food passes from the mouth and esophagus (hence,

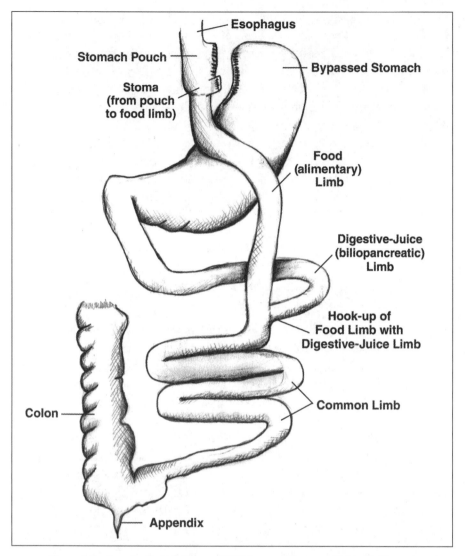

Figure 3.2. Regular Gastric Bypass (GBP) Surgery (Roux-en-Y Gastric Bypass)

the *food limb,* or *alimentary limb*). The other slanted limb is the digestive-juice limb, medically termed the *biliopancreatic limb* because bile and pancreatic digestive juices pass through it. The bypassed stomach empties into this limb. The food limb and the digestive juice limb meet at the central crotch of the "Y." This is where the digestive juices flowing from one limb begin to mix with and digest the food from the other limb, as they empty together into the common limb, the vertical, lower part of the "Y." Normally, once it has mixed with, and is digested by, the digestive juices, most of the food is then absorbed through the walls of the common limb into the body. The remaining unabsorbed food and liquids then pass out of the common limb into the large intestine and, thereafter, out through the rectum and anus.

The digestive juice limb carries acid and other digestive juices from the bypassed stomach, bile from the liver, and digestive juices from the pancreas and the lining of the bypassed small intestines. These juices assist in the digestion and absorption of food. Instead of mixing with food in the previously large stomach, these juices now inefficiently mix with the food lower down in the intestines, so that less of the swallowed food and liquid is digested and absorbed. This results in malabsorption, where the unabsorbed food is "lost" to the body in the stool.

There are variations of gastric bypass surgery that are meant to enhance weight loss. These are discussed below.

Extended Gastric Bypass (X–GBP)

Some surgeons shorten or lengthen the limbs in the Roux-en-Y in various ways. For example, some surgeons form a 3-foot-long food limb and a 7-foot-long common limb, with the rest of the intestines being bypassed as the digestive-juice limb. Other surgeons do just the opposite. In procedures where the food limb is lengthened beyond 5 feet, the surgery may be

Potential Complications Associated With Weight-Loss Surgery

Potential problems associated with bariatric surgery include those seen after any surgery on the abdomen such as wound infection, heart or lung problems, intestinal obstruction (sometimes called *locked bowels*), as well as ventral hernias or blood clots (deep venous thrombosis) that may travel to the lungs (pulmonary embolus), possibly resulting in death. Weight-loss surgery procedures may have any of these complications or specific complications, such as a leak from a staple line, an abnormally narrowed or ulcerated stomach pouch, protein malnutrition, anemia, vitamin/mineral deficiencies, and digestive problems. Moreover, the changes in brain chemistry that occur during massive weight loss can result in varying degrees of depression in about 20 percent of the people who undergo bariatric surgery.

described as a *long limb GBP,* or *extended gastric bypass (X-GBP).* These measures are taken to produce more malabsorption than that achieved with the regular GBP and, therefore, produce more weight loss with even greater improvement in comorbidities. Your surgeon should be able to provide you with more detail about the particular variation(s) of the GBP that he performs as well as its projected weight-loss results. However, the more malabsorption each procedure produces, the greater the risk that malnutrition may develop over the long term.

Super-morbidly obese people—that is, those with BMIs greater than 50—tend to choose X-GBP, since they have so much more weight to lose than the average qualifying patient. These procedures are certainly more effective for their purposes, but the greater the benefit, the more risk there is.

The nutritional problems that arise from X-GBP, as well as from all other forms of malabsorptive surgeries, are quite similar. Just as mentioned above with the super-morbidly obese, the differences arise largely as a matter of risk. That is, nutritional problems are more likely to arise with malabsorptive procedures, and, the more malabsorptive the procedure, the greater the likelihood, as well as severity, of the complications that may occur.

The Banded Gastric Bypass

The banded gastric bypass is a combination of the gastric bypass and the vertical banded gastroplasty. In this procedure, sometimes called the *Fobi, Capella, Fobi-Capella,* or *Memphis bypass* procedure, a band is commonly placed around, or just below, the middle of the stomach pouch. Since the restrictive effects of a banded gastric bypass last longer than do those of a non-banded pouch, which may stretch over time, it has become increasingly popular with some surgeons and their patients. People select this surgery especially when they want to be reasonably sure that the weight loss from their regular GBP will continue long term. In some cases, people who have had a regular gastric bypass opt to have a band added at some later time. Many of our patients who chose to undergo this additional procedure have lost an additional fifteen to forty pounds. However, this procedure involves adding more restriction to the usual gastric bypass. Therefore, those who have it are more likely to experience nausea and vomiting than those who have unrestricted bypass procedures.

The Biliopancreatic Diversion (BPD)

Two other variations of the GBP leave a considerably larger stomach pouch than other surgeries. Developed more than twenty-five years ago, the biliopancreatic diversion (BPD) involves making a much shorter common limb (twenty inches) and a longer food limb (six and two-thirds feet) than the regular gastric bypass. About three-quarters of the stomach are removed, leaving a large stomach pouch, about 10 ounces in size. This allows a person to swallow a lot more food at one time than with the regular gastric bypass. However, the twenty-inch-long common limb is too short to absorb all of this food. This results in large, frequent bowel movements, the potential for dumping syndrome (see page 48), and a risk of malnutrition if the patient does not eat sufficient food and liquids for his needs. Some surgeons, like us, are more conservative, and fashion a common limb that is twice as long (about forty inches) in order to reduce malnutrition risks.

Mild, moderate, or severe malnutrition may occur in about 10 to 20 percent of BPD patients. This is usually related to frequent liquid bowel movements that result in a large loss of protein, salt, water, vitamins, minerals, or other nutrients. Fortunately, such problems are usually controlled with medications and careful food selection.

This procedure is popular with those who do not want to be as limited in their food intake as other weight-loss-surgery patients and yet lose as much weight, if not more, than any other type of bariatric surgery (approximately 80 percent). Also attractive about the BPD is that nausea and vomiting are uncommon when compared with other types of bariatric surgery.

The BPD-Duodenal Switch (BPD-DS)

The BPD-duodenal switch (BPD-DS) is a variation of the BPD. In this surgery, all but a long stapled tube of the lesser curve of the stomach is removed (see Figure 3.3 on page 49). This stomach tube runs from the point at which the esophagus joins the stomach to the muscular valve at the bottom of the stomach called the *pylorus*. The small intestine is divided about 2 inches below the pylorus with surgical staples and the same length (six-and-two-thirds feet) food limb is attached there, all limb lengths being the same as in the BPD. The main reported advantage of this surgery is that people do not experience dumping syndrome (see page 48) and, therefore, are less likely to become malnourished. Also attractive to many people is the fact that, like the BPD, about three-quarters of them lose approximately 80 percent of their excess body weight.

NEWER SURGERIES AND APPROACHES

New surgical procedures or variations or rebirths of old ones regularly arise; some work and others don't. Weight-loss surgery is no exception.

Dumping Syndrome

Dumping syndrome, also called *rapid gastric emptying,* occurs when swallowed food and liquids pass so rapidly to the rectum that the person has little warning and cannot make it to a restroom in time. While more frequent in the BPD, it can occur in any of the variations of the gastric bypass. Another form of this condition occurs when the swallowed food and liquid (often containing a large amount of sugar) passes right into the small intestine from the stomach pouch and is rapidly absorbed into the body. The sugar raises blood sugar levels so quickly that the person's heart rate increases, he feels faint, and his face becomes flushed. This is usually short lived but sometimes may be associated with an urgent need to visit the restroom. In unusual cases, these problems may occur many times each day and result in malnutrition.

Therefore, we advise extreme caution when considering "new" or "better" weight-loss surgery operations that are not well accepted by the vast majority of obesity surgeons. Any person who opts for such a surgery is taking a leap of faith and putting himself at a higher risk than necessary when compared with today's well-accepted, effective, and relatively safe weight-loss-surgery procedures.

Some of the newer surgical approaches do appear promising, however. One such approach is called a *staged operation.* That is, the surgeon performs part of the surgery as a first stage with the intention of helping the person lose some weight. Later, the surgeon performs the second half of the surgery on this lighter and therefore less-risky patient.

Staging of the duodenal switch and of the gastric bypass are two examples of newer, but not completely proven, procedures. Performing the duodenal switch in two steps may be useful in cases of super-morbidly obese people who also have additional medical problems that make them too high a risk for the complete duodenal switch procedure.

An intriguing possibility that is now being reported internationally is to use the adjustable gastric band as a first stage of a gastric bypass. Later, instead of staples, the band is inflated so that it completely closes off the upper stomach to make a pouch. Then, a small intestinal Roux-en-Y is made, and the upper end of the food limb is attached to the pouch. The adjustable gastric band may be inflated during surgery or later. A significant advantage of this procedure is that the inflatable band can easily be deflat-

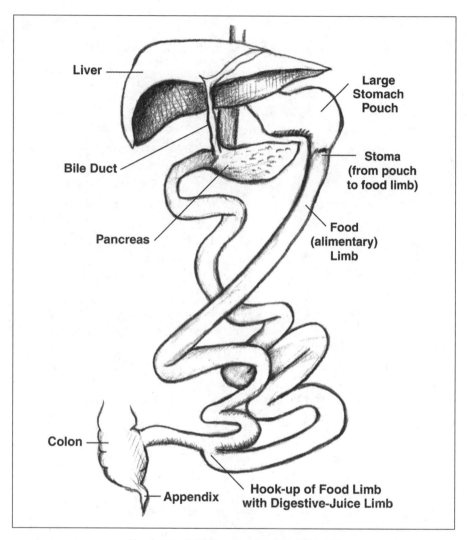

Figure 3.3.   BPD-Duodenal Switch (BPD-DS)

ed at any time in case of complications. And, of course, with fewer or no staple lines, there is less risk of developing a leak. However, it is possible that the inflated band may hold the stomach so tightly that it winds up eroding through the stomach wall, thereby producing serious complications months or even years following the surgery. It's too soon to know exactly what the long-term outcome will be. Until good outcomes have been reported with at least five years of follow-up, we do not recommend this procedure as part of a gastric bypass to our patients .

Future Alternatives to Weight-Loss Surgery

As it stands today, about 95 percent of all morbidly obese people fail at their long-term efforts to lose and keep off excess weight non-surgically. Currently, weight-loss surgery has proven itself to be the best solution for long-term weight loss. This doesn't mean, however, that the future doesn't hold promise for alternative treatments. Research into fat storage and obesity has made major strides in the past few years. A full scientific understanding of how the human body works with regard to fat storage, hunger messages, satiety, and the like may eventually lead to successful non-surgical treatments. In the meantime, there are a lot of unanswered questions. For instance, how does the body keep track of, or manage, its contents—fat, protein, minerals, sugar, and so on? Another question along these lines is, what drives the body and its owner to eat and store fat up to a given level? Various theories are emerging, but at this time we have no solid answers.

Almost all morbidly obese people are physically unable to feel full from the food and drink they consume. It is thought that their bodies are defective in some way that prevents them from feeling satisfied. This may be due to faulty nerves in the stomach that fail to register the "full" feeling when an adequate amount of food has been eaten. Alternatively, hormones that are released from the stomach and intestines may fail to relay messages of fullness to the brain. Or perhaps the brain itself cannot properly recognize these messages or maybe the defect lies in the nerve pathways themselves. Obviously, the challenge here is to find out where the defect is and to figure out how fix it.

There are many other parts to this complex puzzle of what causes obesity and how to cure it, including the genetic link. Researchers are currently investigating many candidate genes that may be responsible for obesity. Although we know a lot of things about many pieces of this puzzle, our view of the real cause or causes of obesity remains unclear.

What's clear is that, at this time, weight-loss surgery is the only way for the vast majority of morbidly obese people to lose massive amounts of weight and keep it off for life. Of course, as time wears on, weight-loss surgery itself should become more effective and less risky with fewer potential complications and side effects. This, of course, is good news for everyone involved. Weight-loss surgery should also become less expensive and more routine, benefiting a larger majority of people.

While it's true that a lot questions remain unanswered at this time, research is ongoing, and the answers are bound to be discovered. We anticipate major breakthroughs in the next thirty to sixty years in our scientific understanding of what causes obesity, resulting in an effective non-surgical means of controlling excess weight. Until then, weight-loss surgery is offered as a potentially available, invaluable, and proven aid in improving your health.

A number of other surgical possibilities may become available to help manage morbid obesity within the next few years. For instance, it is likely that new-and-improved gastric bands will be approved by the U.S. Food and Drug Administration (FDA) in the near future; some of these bands are already being used in Europe and elsewhere. The newer bands are designed to have fewer complications involving band migration, erosion, obstruction, leakage, or other problems. Long-term results are needed, however.

Another possible weight-loss surgery being studied is the gastric pacemaker for weight loss. Like a pacemaker that's used to control the heart's rhythm, a pacemaker electrode is laparoscopically implanted into the stomach wall to electrically stimulate, or pace, the stomach in an effort to make a person want to eat less. An electrode is attached to a wire connected to a battery pack and a computer chip sewn under the skin and fat on the front of the abdomen. The stimulator sends programmed electrical impulses to the stomach pacemaker wire and reads electrical messages from the stomach wall. This device is currently under consideration for FDA approval. Weight-loss results from gastric pacemaker studies have been somewhat on the low side, but, with more research, they may improve.

OTHER PROCEDURES COMMONLY PERFORMED DURING WEIGHT-LOSS SURGERY

It is often necessary or beneficial for a person to undergo additional procedures during weight-loss surgery. The most common of these include gastrostomy tube insertion, gallbladder removal, hiatus hernia repair, ventral hernia repair, liver biopsy, tummy tuck, tubal ligation, and ovarian cyst removal. Each of these procedures is discussed below.

Gastrostomy Tube (G–Tube) Insertion

Following weight-loss surgery, the bypassed stomach continues to make acid, mucus, and other digestive juices. If the pylorus, the muscular valve at the bottom of the stomach, should spasm, the stomach may not empty these juices. As a result, it can stretch out and inflate like a balloon so much that it bursts, thereby causing a leak, an increased heart rate, and a serious drop in blood pressure, among other problems. Therefore, some surgeons regularly place a drainage tube, called a *gastrostomy tube* (G-tube), into the bypassed stomach. Other surgeons do so only with certain patients who they think may develop this type of drainage problem. Other surgeons, especially laparoscopists, rarely use a drainage tube. In other words, the use of the G-tube depends upon a surgeon's experience, judgment, and whether he performs open or laparoscopic weight-loss surgery.

When left open, the G-tube acts like a pressure valve on a pressure kettle. It allows the extra juices to pass out of the bypassed stomach when the pylorus is in spasm. Also, in cases where a person has difficulty taking food or medications, particularly in the case of severe diabetes, this tube can be used to provide liquids until the patient is able to swallow medications and food once again.

Gallbladder Removal

Nearly one-third of weight-loss-surgery patients have had their gallbladders removed prior to the surgery. If a person still has his gallbladder at the time of surgery, there's a good chance an abnormality will be present. (According to reports, a gallbladder abnormality exists in about 95 percent of obese patients.) Therefore, some surgeons recommend gallbladder removal, or a cholecystectomy, during bariatric surgery; it takes about ten minutes in open surgery but up to twice as long, or longer, laparoscopically. Other surgeons do not recommend gallbladder removal because of the extended surgery time and because they have a reasonable doubt that a particular patient will ever experience gallbladder-related problems. However, if a person's history or tests indicate that gallstones are present, it's wise to proceed with gallbladder removal. When the gallbladder remains, massive weight loss may result in the development of gallstones. To help prevent these gallstones, a surgeon may prescribe the bile salt chenodeoxycholic acid, which hinders stone formation, until weight loss levels off.

Hiatus Hernia Repair

Chronic or relatively frequent heartburn, burping, upper abdominal pain, and certain food intolerances are usually symptoms of a hiatus hernia. As explained in Chapter 1, this condition develops when the opening that the esophagus passes through in the diaphragm, called a *hiatus*, becomes abnormally widened, allowing stomach acid to freely pass upward to irritate and inflame the esophagus. By bypassing most of the acid-producing stomach, gastric bypass procedures usually prevent most acid from reaching the esophagus. However, it is possible for some people to produce enough acid even from their small stomach pouches to cause problems. Therefore, some surgeons offer to repair a hiatus hernia during weight-loss surgery. This procedure, called a *hiatal herniorrhaphy*, usually involves an additional five minutes or so to make the esophageal hiatus smaller.

Ventral Hernia Repair

A ventral hernia is a weakness or defect of the abdominal wall through which tissues inside the abdominal cavity protrude abnormally. Hernias do not resolve on their own; repairing them, if necessary, requires surgery. In many cases, a surgeon will repair a preexisting ventral hernia during bariatric surgery. In rare cases, however, a ventral hernia may be too large or too inconvenient to repair during the surgery. Therefore, a surgeon may advise against repairing it until after weight loss has occurred. Such delayed ventral hernia repairs may also be accompanied by a tummy tuck (see page 54).

In other cases, a surgeon may discover a ventral hernia while performing bariatric surgery. Often, this "surprise" ventral hernia, usually small in size, will be repaired when discovered. Unlike the large variety, repair of a small ventral hernia may add only a few minutes to the overall procedure time, since it is usually performed as part of closing up the abdomen. (See the inset "About Ventral Hernias" in Chapter 9 on page 165 for information on ventral hernias that occur after surgery.)

Liver Biopsy

About 95 percent of all morbidly obese people have an abnormality of the liver. In most of these cases, the liver is filled with fat in varying amounts. In some cases, liver cirrhosis (scarring) is present. If a severe case of cirrhosis is discovered at the time of bariatric surgery, the surgeon may choose to discontinue, or modify, the weight-loss operation. This is an individual decision each surgeon may need to make at the time of the surgery. In any case, during surgery, the surgeon may take several minutes to obtain a liver biopsy (a piece of the liver) for later examination under the microscope.

Tummy Tuck

A tummy tuck, medically termed an *abdominoplasty*, is a surgical procedure in which excess skin and fat are removed from the lower abdomen. People usually opt to have this surgery and other types of cosmetic surgery after they've lost their excess weight. However, some surgeons offer their patients the option of having a tummy tuck during the bariatric surgery itself. This procedure adds at least an hour or more to the time required for the surgery. Moreover, instead of a 1 to 2 percent chance of developing a wound infection, a person who has a tummy tuck during bariatric surgery has a 10 percent or so chance of developing an infection. Many surgeons do not offer this combined procedure; when it is offered, however, it is up to the individual to decide whether to take the additional risks involved. (See Chapter 11 for more on cosmetic surgery.)

Tubal Ligation and Cyst Removal

If prearranged with the surgeon, a female patient who does not wish to become pregnant can have her Fallopian tubes surgically divided during bariatric surgery to prevent pregnancy. This procedure, called *tubal ligation*, will add about ten minutes or so to the surgery; however, if adhesions or other problems are present, it may take longer.

In some cases, during surgery, a surgeon may discover and remove cysts on the ovaries. Some medical professionals believe that cyst removal may help previously infertile patients to become more likely to conceive in the future.

A hysterectomy, the removal of the uterus, with or without the Fallopian tubes and ovaries is a major surgery in itself; therefore, it's advisable to avoid or defer this procedure until a later time.

CONCLUSION

This chapter has familiarized you with the surgical options that may be available to you. It's also given you some idea about what goes on during surgery. Your surgeon will generally recommend a certain surgery, which will most likely be the one he has had the most success with. Learn as much as you can about the recommended surgery and don't hesitate to ask about other possibilities.

Now that you know whether or not you're likely to qualify for surgery and what types of weight-loss surgeries are available, you're ready to make some decisions. The next chapter will help you on your way.

$\mathcal{M}$AKING AND SHARING YOUR DECISION

n times past, surgeons were the decision-makers. They told their patients what surgeries they were going to perform, and the patients rarely objected or asked questions about the surgery. In other words, they gave the surgeons their blind consent. This is no longer the case. These days, surgeons are partners in the decision-making process, especially when it involves elective or planned surgery. You should expect a potential surgeon to take the time to discuss your options with you as well as the details of the surgery you are considering. You and, often, your family members should receive the necessary information to help you decide whether or not to have the surgery.

In order to reach the point where your mind is made up, you need to know what weight-loss surgery is all about. The learning process should begin from the moment you hear about the surgery and continue until you place your signature on the "Informed Consent" form. Legally speaking, this document acknowledges that you fully understand the procedure(s) to be performed as well as the alternatives, who is doing the surgery, what the risks are, what the benefits are, and what possible complications might occur. Unlike those patients from the past, you are not merely told what your surgery will be, and you certainly are not expected to give your blind consent. Your consent should be well informed.

Although you don't need to be an expert in every detail of the surgery, you do need to know where you can find the information you desire. You also need to know the right questions to ask. The answers should give you enough information to enable you to make up your mind about whether a certain operation is right for you and, just as important, who you want to do that surgery. This chapter will help you make those decisions and will provide some suggestions for sharing your decision to have weight-loss surgery with those closest to you.

DISCUSSING WEIGHT-LOSS SURGERY
WITH YOUR PRIMARY-CARE PHYSICIAN (PCP)

When it comes to weight-loss surgery, you can think of your PCP as a gate-keeper. When you ask her to refer you for weight-loss surgery, the answer you receive will be *yes* or *no*. In one case, the PCP swings the gate wide open by giving you a referral to consult with a weight-loss surgeon. In the other case, the "gatekeeper" won't allow you to pass through the gate. In that PCP's opinion, weight-loss surgery is not a good idea for you.

If you strongly disagree with your doctor's opinion, you may wish to find another PCP. This new PCP may be able to help you pass through the gate. However, before you go in search of a new doctor, you need to clear-ly understand why your PCP has taken this position. Ask your doctor to explain why she doesn't think weight-loss surgery is right for you. If her points are reasonable, you might want to abide by the decision.

PCPs are not experts in weight-loss surgery, but many are familiar with the basics. Some have seen excellent results in their patients who have had weight-loss surgery. Unfortunately, others have been witness to serious complications, particularly in the earlier days when the surgery was risk-ier. This, of course, will affect the way they view the surgery as well as the advice they give you. If your PCP is simply against weight-loss surgery for any reason, at any cost, you might want to consider finding a new, more open-minded doctor.

What you really want to know from your PCP is, in her professional judgment, will weight-loss surgery be worth it for you? For instance, your PCP will calculate your BMI to see if you are large enough to qualify. She will also determine if you are sick enough (or well enough) to seriously consider the surgery. If you are not completely familiar with the details of your health, be sure to learn from your PCP precisely what your health problems are. Then, with your current health in mind, ask your doctor if she thinks surgery is worth it. If, after taking all the factors into consideration, your PCP thinks you should pursue weight-loss surgery, she may be able to recommend a good surgeon.

While you're at your PCP's office, keep in mind that the weight-loss surgeon's office will need certain details from your health record to clear you for surgery. You can't be expected to remember every detail of your health history, so be sure to ask your PCP for any relevant information in your file. Your PCP can provide you or your surgeon or other members of the health-care team with copies of your recent lab results and any other relevant studies for review. Your PCP may want to perform some additional tests before giving you a referral. It's a good idea to make sure your health-insurance provider will cover these additional tests.

Once your PCP gives you the referral, it's time to make an appointment to see a weight-loss surgeon.

FINDING A WEIGHT-LOSS SURGEON

After reading Chapter 3, you probably have some idea which type of weight-loss surgery you'd be most comfortable having. If you do have a specific surgery in mind, you'll need to find a surgeon who performs it. Not every weight-loss surgeon, or *bariatric surgeon*, performs every type of surgery. A surgeon may perform only one or two particular operations because those are the surgeries that work best in her hands and with her patients. Other surgeons may provide a wider range of surgeries and will try to match patients to a surgery that they believe will be best for them.

Locating Weight-Loss Surgeons in Your Area

Your PCP may be familiar with some of the surgeons who perform weight-loss surgery in or near your community and might give you a good recommendation. However, since PCPs have such a wide range of specialties to deal with, they might be underinformed in a particular area, including this one. Therefore, it will be up to you to locate the surgeon in your area who is right for you.

You can begin your search by attending a meeting of a weight-loss-surgery support group. These groups are patient-centered, and, as part of the program, members usually share their personal experiences with the rest of the group. Some of these people speak freely about their experiences with weight-loss surgery, both good and bad. You can ask group members if they are happy with their results, and if you get some mixed messages, you may want to attend another surgeon's support-group meeting. There is nothing wrong with "checking out the field." (There's more on the benefits of attending weight-loss-surgery support groups in Chapter 5.)

The Internet can provide you with a number of possible leads if other sources don't turn up anything. Be aware, however, that simply typing key words such as "bariatric surgery" into a search engine will turn up hundreds of thousands of results. While there will be many reputable sites among them, such as the site for the American Society for Bariatric Surgery

(ASBS), which provides an extensive database of bariatric surgeons, there are many others you should steer clear of. For instance, we strongly recommend that you avoid any websites, as well as the surgeons affiliated with them, that offer outdated or experimental surgeries.

If you find a surgeon in your area through a link to her website, you can search for that surgeon on the ASBS website database (see the Resources section) to determine her membership in the organization. If she is a regular member of the ASBS, board certification or at least eligibility for board certification is certain. And that, of course, is a good starting point when selecting a surgeon. Additionally, you will want to note whether the surgeon and her hospital have been designated as an "ASBS Bariatric Surgery Center of Excellence" by the ASBS Surgical Review Corporation. The ASBS website lists these centers by state and city.

During your Internet search, you may come across links to weight-loss-surgery support groups. Keep in mind that while these groups can be helpful for day-to-day coping, you need to locate a reputable and professional source for medical information. (For more advice, see the inset "Sorting Out the Good From the Bad on the Internet" on page 90 in Chapter 5.)

Familiarizing Yourself With Potential Surgeons

When you have a few names of surgeons in your area, you'll need to contact them for further information. If you have the surgeon's e-mail address, you can send a note by e-mail. Otherwise, call the surgeon's office directly.

Find out what type of program the surgeon offers. Ask if she has a support group. If so, find out when and where it meets, and plan to attend. Most bariatric surgeons also give lectures or seminars periodically. If the surgeon you're interested in is offering a lecture or seminar, be sure to attend. This way, you can hear what the surgeon has to offer in a group setting without committing yourself to anything. Almost all meetings of this type are open to the public without charge, and you are usually encouraged to bring family or friends along with you.

When you contact a surgeon's office or register for a lecture or meeting, the office may send you some literature for review and/or forms for you to fill out. Or you may receive this information and paperwork during or after the meeting or lecture. Filling out the forms is optional at this stage, so do whatever you feel comfortable doing.

If you cannot make it to a particular surgeon's lecture or seminar, she may offer an audiotape or video recording for you to listen to or watch. Keep in mind that this doesn't give you the chance to participate in the question-and-answer part of the lecture or seminar. There is nothing quite like being there to "get a feel" for the people giving the lectures, which, of course, may give you a better feel for the surgeon and her program.

Choosing Among Surgeons

An important part of choosing a surgeon is learning as much as you can about her experience with weight-loss surgery and to keep a record of it so that you can compare notes on different surgeons. Start by answering the following yes-or-no questions for each surgeon you are considering. In some cases, this information will be available in the surgeon's literature; in other cases, the surgeon will communicate this information to you as a matter of course. If not, you'll have to ask for the information.

1. Is the surgeon board certified or at least board eligible by the American Board of Surgery as a general surgeon?

2. Have you met the surgeon? If so, does she seem like the kind of person with whom you feel comfortable and confident?

3. Has the surgeon's office staff treated you kindly and with respect?

4. Does the surgeon provide a booklet or other literature that clearly describes her weight-loss-surgery program?

5. Does it seem like a good program for both before and after the surgery?

6. Is periodic consultation with a dietician or nutritionist part of the post-surgery program?

7. Is there an active, well-attended support group for the surgeon's patients?

8. Does the surgeon offer one-on-one mental health support with an experienced therapist and/or treatment when necessary?

9. Are you confident that the surgeon and the surgeon's staff are dedicated to helping you—not only now, but also five or ten years from now?

10. As part of the surgeon's program, are you expected to return periodically for checkups for the rest of your life?

Obviously, you'll want to answer "yes" to most of the above questions. If you've received satisfactory answers, have the surgeon answer the questions in the "Bariatric Surgeon Questionnaire" on page 60. Comparing

Bariatric Surgeon Questionnaire

1. How many years have you been performing bariatric
   surgery?   _____

2. How many bariatric surgeries have you performed?   _____

3. How many bariatric surgeries have you performed
   in the past year?   _____

4. Which type of surgical approach do you recommend for me:
   ❏ Open bariatric surgery
   ❏ Laparoscopic bariatric surgery
   And why do you recommend it?

   _____

   _____

   *How many of the recommended type of surgery
   have you done in total?*   _____

   *How many of the recommended type of surgery
   have you done in the past year?*   _____

5. Exactly which procedure do you propose for me?

   _____

   _____

   How many of these procedures have you done in total?   _____

   *How many of these procedures have you done in
   the past year?*   _____

6. On average, how many hours does it take you to
   perform this procedure?   _____

7. Is the surgery you propose for me a type of surgery
   that most weight-loss surgeons perform?   _____

If the answer is no, ask what makes this surgery different from the surgeries that most other weight-loss surgeons perform. Also, ask how long this type of surgery has been around and how long this surgeon has been performing it. Also, ask the following two questions:

7a. Is this surgery experimental?   _____

7b. What are the possible complications and what is the likelihood of their occurrence in your experience? How does this compare with others?

_____

_____

8. For any of the bariatric surgeries—especially the one proposed for you—ask:

What is the average weight loss and time frame associated with this surgery?   _____   _____

What is the range of this weight loss, lowest to highest?   _____ – _____

What is the average percentage of excess body weight lost?   _____

What is the range from lowest to highest?   _____ – _____

9. What percentage of your patients have died following weight-loss surgery?   _____

What percentage of your patients have died in the past year following weight-loss surgery?   _____

What was the cause of death?

_____

10. What percentage of your patients have had serious complications after weight-loss surgery?   _____

What were the complications?

_____

_____

answers from different surgeons will help you choose among them. Since there is no one correct answer, be sure to compare the information you receive very carefully in light of the information in the book and specifically in the section "Interpreting the Results of the Questionnaire" below. Having this information and knowing what it implies should help you make the right decision.

If a surgeon refuses to or does not wish to answer your questions, you have the right to seek someone else who will provide you with the information you need to make an informed decision. Having access to all of this information is an important part of the informed-consent process and should be made available to you before you sign any documents permitting a surgeon to perform weight-loss surgery on you.

Interpreting the Results of the Questionnaire

Review the surgeon's answers and compare them to the following numbered items. (Numbered items below correspond to the numbered questions in the questionnaire.)

1. A surgeon's experience performing bariatric surgery is a very important factor to take into consideration during the selection process. A surgeon who has had many years' experience with weight-loss surgery will be more familiar and better able to deal with most of the major complications than a surgeon who has less experience. (See also the discussion on question 4 for more about a surgeon's experience performing laparoscopic surgery.)

2. Theoretically, each time a person performs a task, the better she becomes at carrying it out. The number of tries it takes to do that task skillfully (the learning curve) depends on the task being preformed. In general, the learning curve for *open* weight-loss surgery is thirty to fifty surgeries. Therefore, unless you are willing to be operated on by a surgeon who is, in essence, still learning, you'll want to choose a surgeon who has performed more than fifty of these surgeries. For *laparoscopic* weight-loss surgery, the learning curve extends to at least the first one hundred or so surgeries. (These cases can include the laparoscopic surgeries the surgeon performed as part of her training.)

3. In addition to the *total* number of surgeries a surgeon has performed, the *annual* number of surgeries she performs is also an important consideration. Research indicates that the patients of surgeons who perform at least seventy-five surgeries a year have fewer complications and other surgery-related problems than the patients of surgeons who do not meet this annu-al minimum. Therefore, if you choose a surgeon who performs seventy-five or more cases per year, your risks of experiencing a major complication *should* be lower.

4. Why should you be concerned about a surgeon's experience performing laparoscopic bariatric surgery specifically? The recent popularity of weight-loss surgery and laparoscopic surgical techniques has prompted many gen-eral surgeons to take weight-loss surgery courses and begin performing laparoscopic bariatric surgery. Therefore, you may encounter many sur-geons who may have taken laparoscopic courses recently but have little actual laparoscopic weight-loss surgical experience. If you cannot find a surgeon who has an acceptable amount of experience performing laparo-scopic bariatric surgery, your best option is to undergo open bariatric sur-gery with a surgeon who is experienced in that area. Be sure to choose a surgeon with adequate experience to fully understand the complexities that occur with the particular procedure you wish to have.

5. A weight-loss surgeon should provide you with a complete description of the operation she proposes for you. This is particularly important for moderately or severely malabsorptive procedures. Record the proposed length of the food limb and common limb and compare them to the stan-dard lengths discussed in Chapter 3.

6. Even in experienced hands, open bariatric surgery often takes longer than laparoscopic bariatric surgery. The average operating time for open surgery is usually under three hours, preferably two. However, in cases of super-morbidly obese patients (that is, patients with a BMI of 50 or higher), up to one hour or so may be needed to securely close up the abdomen. In that case, an average of three hours is acceptable. Keep in mind that extra time may be required to perform additional surgeries, such as gallbladder removal and liver biopsy. (Additional procedures that may be performed immediately following weight-loss surgery are discussed in Chapter 3.)

Early in most laparoscopic surgeons' experience, the first few surgeries performed may take up to five or more hours. As a surgeon gains more experience, the operation can be performed quicker, usually within one to three hours.

7. It's wise to avoid, or at least very closely evaluate, any weight-loss pro-cedure that is relatively new or experimental. Before recommending a pro-cedure, we generally like to see that it has had successful long-term results (five years or more). If only short-term results are available for a particular procedure, greater risks, some still unknown, may be involved.

If a surgeon recommends a type of weight-loss surgery not described in Chapter 3, it is very likely experimental at the time of this publication. For instance, a gastric bypass operation without the Roux-en-Y (see Chapter 3) is unacceptable to most weight-loss surgeons; if it is presented to you as an option, it would be best to not even consider it.

Also, if your surgeon recommends a moderate to severe type of malabsorptive surgery, you'll want to know what percentage of her patients has problems, such as diarrhea and malnutrition. Moreover, you'll want to know what percentage of the surgeon's patients who had the surgery she proposes for you needed to repeat the surgery and why. For example, if 20 percent of a surgeon's patients needed reoperation, you'd probably want to avoid this procedure; 20 percent is rather high. However, by today's standard, 5 percent is acceptable. Carefully consider anything higher than that.

The National Institutes of Health has established weight-loss-surgery centers around the country in which to study the various surgeries and related benefits. In time, we'll have more comprehensive information regarding the pros and cons of each surgery. For now, the information presented in this book is as complete as it can be. If you are still in doubt about your choices, reread Chapter 3.

8. How much weight a person is likely to lose depends a lot on her starting weight and the type of surgery she has. There are many factors to take into consideration, too many, in fact, to cover them all here. Therefore, discussing the weight-loss potential associated with various surgeries with your surgeon is very important.

Here's an example to give you some idea what the numbers will mean to you. If a woman with an ideal body weight of 150 pounds weighs 250 pounds, she would need to lose about 100 pounds to reach her ideal weight. If she weighs 350 pounds, however, she would need to lose about 200 pounds. Since most restrictive procedures average less than 100 pounds of total weight loss, a person with more weight to lose would likely choose a gastric bypass Roux-en-Y, which is associated with a higher average weight loss. While a 250-pound person could go with either type of surgery, she would be wise to think twice before undergoing a severe malabsorptive procedure since she could potentially lose *too much* weight.

When looking at the percentages of how much excess weight is lost with a particular surgery, be sure to take the starting weights into consideration. For example, compare the 350-pound person's weight loss of 100 pounds with the 250-pound person's weight loss of the same amount. The 350-pound person will have lost only half, or 50 percent, of her excess body weight while the 250-pound person will have lost all, or 100 percent, of her excess weight. This is why it is important to consider all the numbers, especially the relationship between your actual weight and your ideal body weight. (See the inset "What's Your Ideal Body Weight" below.)

9. Death rates vary and depend on various factors, including how many high-risk patients a surgeon operates on. For example, a surgeon who operates on patients with an average BMI of 60 will have a higher death rate associated with her practice than a surgeon who does not operate on anyone with a BMI higher than 50 because of the higher risks involved. In any event, the average death rate most often quoted in bariatric-surgery literature is 0.5 percent. This equals one death for every two hundred patients a surgeon has operated on. A figure lower than 1 percent is generally considered acceptable. However, quality surgeons who perform surgery on higher-risk patients may have a figure somewhat greater than 1 percent, and this may be considered acceptable.

One-third to one-half of the deaths that occur after weight-loss surgery

---

What's Your Ideal Body Weight?

If you don't have access to an ideal body weight chart, you can still get a pretty good idea of what your ideal body weight is with the following figures.

For Women

1. Start with a base figure of 100 pounds at a height of 5 feet.
2. For every inch above or below this height, add or subtract 5 pounds. (When dealing with half inches, round up to the nearest inch.)

    For example, if you are 5 feet 5 inches tall, your approximate ideal body weight would be 125 pounds. That is, 100 pounds + 5 x 5 = 125.

For Men

1. Start with a base figure of 110 pounds at a height of 5 feet.
2. For every inch above or below this height, add or subtract 6 pounds. (When dealing with half inches, round up to the nearest inch.)

    For example, if you are 5 feet 5 inches tall, your approximate ideal body weight would be 140 pounds. That is, 110 pounds + 6 x 5 = 140.

Does My Mind Have to Be Made Up
Before I Contact a Surgeon?

Although it's not a requirement, most weight-loss surgeons prefer that a person has made up her mind at least reasonably well that she wants weight-loss surgery by the time she comes to their office for a history and physical examination. Of course, this is not absolutely necessary. They, and you, must understand that you have the absolute right to decide against having the surgery up to the time you are anesthetized on the operating-room table. You are, and must remain, in charge of any decision concerning any procedure to be performed on your body, including weight-loss surgery. That's the law.

are due to clots that partly or completely block the blood vessels leading to the lungs. This is called a *pulmonary embolism.* If this complication occurs, it is frequently fatal. To try to prevent these blood clots from forming, patients are often required to wear special inflatable boots on their feet and legs during and after surgery and may also receive injections of blood thinner. Another main cause of death related to weight-loss surgery is caused by infection and related complications due to leakage from the site of surgical stapling or suturing. (Much less frequently, leakage can occur from dissection around the stomach or intestines.)

10. As you now know, complications can occur with any type of surgery. The surgeon should clearly discuss any possible complications with you. If the surgeon doesn't provide you with her percentage (or numbers) of serious complications, you have every right to ask for this information or look elsewhere.

DISCUSSING YOUR DECISION
TO HAVE WEIGHT-LOSS SURGERY WITH OTHERS

Up until now, you may have been keeping the prospect of having weight-loss surgery to yourself. That's okay during the early stages, but now you need to consider sharing your plans with your family, friends, and colleagues. While you're recovering from your surgery, you will need the active support of at least one or two people you can rely on. It's very important that you discuss all of your plans with them. We'll cover some specifics regarding your support people in the next chapter. For now, however, let's put the focus on sharing your decision with those closest to you in general.

Some people have difficulty telling their families, and, possibly, their friends and coworkers that they are strongly considering, or have already decided upon having, weight-loss surgery. You may be one of those people. However, it's important to understand that, at the very least, your closest family members or friends have a right to know about the surgery so that they, too, can be prepared for what's to come. Also, they'll probably want to know what they can do to help you along in the process. Be sure to give them a copy of this book and earmark certain sections for careful reading, especially Part Four.

In some cases, people keep everything from their families and friends almost until the day of surgery or failed to tell anyone at all. Once again, we strongly recommend against this. Such people usually claim that those closest to them will be against the surgery and they don't want to be talked out of it or made to feel like they are doing the wrong thing. These are not unreasonable concerns. However, trust is an important factor in any relationship. If you want to be trusted by your family members or close friends, you need to start by being open and honest, especially in the face of surgery. Keeping secrets and lying sow the seeds of distrust. Whenever possible, openness is always best.

Having gotten this far in the book, you've invested a good deal of your time learning about weight-loss surgery. When you tell your family or friends about your plans, they'll need and want to know more about the surgery as well, perhaps even before giving you their support. After all, these are the people who love and care about you. It's not unreasonable for them to feel uneasy about any major steps you are going to take to change your life.

Keep in mind that the people in your life may know close to nothing about weight-loss surgery. It's your job to get them informed or to clear up any misconceptions they may have. For instance, it's possible they've heard "bad stories" about the surgery and may fear that you'll die from complications. Remind them that bad news travels faster and farther than good news. Moreover, such stories usually become distorted as they are passed from person to person. Therefore, many of these word-of-mouth tales are sometimes untrue or seriously in error. And, often when they are true, they are referring to older types of weight-loss surgery that are no longer performed due to serious problems. While it's true that every form of surgery has associated complications, one case—particularly a distorted one—does not provide anyone with enough information to decide if a type of surgery is good or bad. If your family members or friends try to base their argument not to have the surgery on a few stories of "surgery gone bad," tell them that there is much more for them to learn and help them get the information they need.

So how do you go about informing your family or close friends about your decision? For starters, begin by explaining how difficult it has been for you to permanently lose weight. Most likely, over the years, they've witnessed your repeated successes and failures. Remind them how much time and effort you've spent trying various diets, exercise routines, behavior-modification courses, and weight-loss medications. Tell them just how painful it was each time you failed and then failed again.

Then, tell them that you're seriously considering weight-loss surgery to put an end to your weight problems once and for all. Make sure they know that you've done your research and that you've given the surgery a great deal of thought. At this point, they may ask you to give it "one more try" without surgery. If they do, you might want to tell them that non-surgical weight-loss methods are unsuccessful more than 95 percent of the time over the long term. That "one more try" has a nearly 100 percent chance of failing. You can also tell them that National Institutes of Health has stated that weight-loss surgery is the only proven way for morbidly obese people to successfully control their weight long term.

Talk freely about what it's like to be obese to give them an idea of just how difficult it is to be morbidly obese. You might find it helpful to make a list of all your obesity-related problems—physical, social, and psychological. During your discussion, you can read from this list or use it as a cue card. Let your family or friends know that you don't want to die ten to fifteen years earlier than the average person. Tell them that you don't want to develop more and more obesity-related disorders as you increase in size. If it's true for you, tell them that you're plain sick and tired of being obese and that you just won't take it anymore.

Naturally, your family will be concerned about the risk of death or serious complications. Discuss your current health concerns and comorbidities. Tell them clearly that you are concerned about becoming more ill and that you do not want to die many years sooner than if you were an average weight. They may be comforted to know that the risk of dying from weight-loss surgery is only about half of 1 percent or less, while the risk of dying from the comorbidities of morbid obesity is much worse. While serious complications of the surgery can occur 5 to 10 percent of the time, assure your family that the surgeon who ultimately performs your operation has a good track record of getting her patients through the surgery if a complication does develop. Inform them that you're not alone in your decision—that, every year, about 200,000 people choose to have this type of surgery usually primarily for the purpose of obtaining better health and a longer life than they could otherwise expect.

Your family members may fear the transformation you will go through following surgery. They may say they like you just the way you are and they don't want you to change. While you will certainly change on the outside, reassure them that you will still be the same person on the inside—we are what we are no matter how we appear on the outside. Also, remind them that you will be able to participate in more and more activities with them as you shed your excess weight. Also, tell them that it's likely you'll be around for many more years at your healthier weight than you otherwise would have been. Yes, you may be more self-confident and have a more "can-do" attitude than you did before your surgery, but you as a person will still be "you."

To get them more comfortable with the idea of your having the surgery, you might want to invite a family member or close friend or two to join you at a weight-loss-surgery support group so they can meet people who've had the surgery. If a weight-loss surgeon is giving a lecture, you can attend with a friend or family member or tape the lecture and ask them to listen to it later.

There's a chance that you will be unable to convince your family members or friends that surgery is your best option. While most family members will support you in your decision and will be pleased that you are moving toward increased health and a better quality of life, some people in your life will be opposed to your having surgery despite your best efforts to convince them otherwise. At that point, you'll need to decide whether or not to proceed with the surgery despite their objections. In most cases, your family and friends will understand that it's your place to decide what's best for you. People who love you will probably accept your decision. That's what love and friendship really come down to—unconditional understanding and acceptance. Unfortunately, not every family or group of friends is capable of that. You may experience difficulties in your relationships before and after your surgery. See the inset "Be Aware of Possible Relationship Troubles or Changes After Surgery" on page 70 to familiarize yourself with some common relationship issues.

Be Aware of Possible Relationship Troubles or Changes After Surgery

There's a very good chance that the postsurgical period—your "second chance"—will bring with it a renewal and revitalization of your existing relationships. Some people, however, may not be quite so lucky. It is for those people that we discuss the following.

While it's true that you will still be the same person you were before the surgery, people may perceive you differently once you've lost your excess weight. Although this altered perception can strengthen some relationships, it can also cause some trouble. It's useful to be aware of what effects weight loss can have on your relationships, as you make your decision to have surgery.

If some of the people closest to you are also overweight or obese, such as a brother or sister, they may become uncomfortable around you once you start losing weight. (Sibling rivalry, unfortunately, doesn't end with childhood.) Other family members or friends might have a difficult time accepting that you've given up your traditional role, perhaps as the caretaker or jokester in the group. Don't be surprised by these attitudes. Instead, prepare yourself ahead of time.

Also, there's a good chance you may lose some of the friends you had

Discussing Surgery With Your Boss and Coworkers

The Health Insurance Portability & Accountability Act (HIPAA) of 1996 gives you the right to withhold details of your personal medical history from others, including your employer. This means that you do not have to tell your boss what type of surgery you're having when you request time off. Whether or not you decide to be specific about the type of surgery you're having depends on the type of relationship you have with your boss. In any event, be sure to give your boss adequate notice and time to make other arrangements, such as hiring a temp during your absence. Depending on the type of surgery you have, you may need as much as a month or two off from work, so be sure to be upfront about this. (It's a good idea to first find out from your surgeon about how much time you'll need to take off, since some procedures do not require such a lengthy recovery period.)

What you decide to tell your coworkers is completely up to you. You should have a pretty good idea of who will cover for you while you're away.

before surgery if your relationship centered on eating together. Companionship based on "food togetherness" will likely fade away after surgery. You'll undoubtedly find things besides eating that attract your interest, and you'll want to spend time engaging in other activities and adventures. This will bring new people, new friends, into your life. That is the natural, expected course of things. As you get smaller, your world will grow larger in many different, beneficial ways.

One relationship that may be affected is your marriage. We have found that on a whole, good marriages get better and bad marriges get worse. For example, Sue's husband was firmly against her having weight-loss surgery. She was sure, however, that he'd be happy with her new look. But after she lost 125 pounds, her husband left her for another woman, an obese woman.

In our experience, some of our female patients' marriages go through a period of separation or end in divorce. For whatever reason, we see this less frequently in the marriages of our male patients. In any event, marriage counseling has often proved useful.

It's important to be aware of these relationship risks when you're making your decision. However, like many others, your relationships may get better with the changes brought on by massive weight loss. (See Chapter 12 for more on your relationships with others.)

Are you concerned that the person or people who must do extra work in your absence will resent you for leaving them with so much work? If you are concerned about having to explain your plans and justify your choice, perhaps it's best to simply say your planned surgery is a private matter. Many of our patients who have chosen to confide in their coworkers report that they were very caring and supportive, and some of them even played an essential role in their support system. You also might find this to be true.

Even if you choose not to disclose to your coworkers the type of surgery you're having, your coworkers will realize that you've gone through something major after you've lost your first fifty to a hundred pounds. Following massive weight loss, many of our patients are no longer worried about sharing the fact that they had weight-loss surgery, since the surgery was obviously a success. At this point, most people volunteer the details of their surgery and take it from there. You may decide to share your plans with your coworkers before your surgery or you may choose to wait until you've had some success. Or you may wish to say nothing at all.

If anyone in your office says you took the easy way out, simply tell that person that it took a lot of courage to have major surgery of any kind, and that includes weight-loss surgery. If you care enough about that person's opinion, give her all the information you gave your friends and family when you first discussed the surgery with them. Your coworker should get the picture of how important and necessary this surgery was for you.

If your coworker still doesn't understand, don't waste any more time on her. There's a good chance you won't have to deal with that person much longer anyway. The majority of our patients get promotions, seek higher education, or interview so well that they land a better job. Chances are that you will have the same type of success.

CONCLUSION

After reading this chapter, you know how important it is to get all the facts, not only about the surgery itself, but also about the surgeon who will ultimately perform your operation, assuming you've decided to move forward. Hopefully, your primary-care physician has given you the go-ahead, you've found a surgeon who you trust, and you've told the people closest to you about your decision to have the surgery. You're on your way!

PART TWO

Your Journey From Presurgery to Recovery

CHAPTER 5

$\mathcal{S}$UPPORT—
AN ESSENTIAL ELEMENT

No matter how independent you are, it's virtually impossible to go through weight-loss surgery alone. Many of the people we see have not leaned on anyone for a long time. Quite often, they are the caretakers not only of themselves but also of their families. To them, asking others for support is truly a foreign concept. Sometimes self-sufficiency has become so much a part of their lives that they have isolated themselves, and, when they look around for help, they find no one. Does this sound like you? If so, to put it quite simply, you *will* need help both before and after the surgery. Hopefully, this chapter will encourage you to seek that help. It will give you some ideas where to look for support, including places you might not have even thought of. Let's take a look at the different avenues available to you.

FINDING SUPPORT IN YOUR SURGEON AND HIS STAFF

You may be surprised to know that one of the key places you'll find support is at your surgeon's office. As you now know, this is not just another routine surgical visit with a quick in and out. The surgeon, as well as the entire staff, will most likely play a much larger part in your life than you had ever imagined. A sensitive and caring surgeon and staff, a knowledgeable team approach, materials provided for your education, and a well-planned program, all have an essential role in your support system, before and after surgery.

Although the surgeon's office may seem like an unusual place to find support, let's take a closer look. This is the first place you may feel genuine care and sensitivity from a medical office. Many people report that their first phone call to a weight-loss surgeon's office was the first time in a long time they felt someone was really listening to them without offering criticism or judgment. That person fully and completely understood not only their myriad medical needs, but also who they were as an individual. This provided initial support by way of kindness, care, and empathy.

Many of you may never have experienced this type of support in a medical office. In fact, as an obese person, you may have come to dread your medical appointments, like Jenny. "I tensed up every time I went to the doctor," Jenny told us. "I knew exactly what would happen. I'd step on the scale and, each and every time, my doctor would say, 'Jenny, you're five-foot-two; you should weigh around a hundred twenty-five pounds. You weigh three hundred pounds. You need to go on a diet.'

"Everything that was wrong with me was blamed on my weight. Usually, no one would listen to anything else. But when I visit my weight-loss surgeon's office, it's a totally different story. I'm usually greeted with a warm hug and a *how are you?* In that office, I know I'm not just another obese person—they *really* want to know how I am. I can feel my body relaxing, and this is just the tip of the iceberg. I actually enjoy going to this doctor's office, because I get the feeling that they care about and understand me, and it makes me feel great!"

In most offices, a surgeon's staff is highly trained and knowledgeable in both the surgery and areas associated with obesity. In fact, the American Society for Bariatric Surgery encourages all support staff members, as well as physicians, to attend conferences, educational events, and meetings. Knowledgeable staff members are available to answer your questions or to clarify anything that may be confusing you, so that you don't have to rely solely on the surgeon. In fact, in many instances throughout this book, we suggest that you call your surgeon for various reasons. Note, however, that your surgeon may not be available to take your call personally. In that case, speaking with a member of the office staff should suffice. And, if necessary, the surgeon will return your call.

Some of the staff members you meet at your surgeon's office might have had the surgery themselves. If so, they will probably be willing to discuss their own experiences. For example, Carol is the front-desk person at a weight-loss surgeon's office. She had weight-loss surgery a while back, and she looks and feels fantastic. When she shares her experience with patients, they are comforted and reassured. They regularly approach her with questions regarding food issues, and she's more than happy to answer them. Carol is a model of life on the other side.

During the presurgical period, you'll quickly learn that, unlike most surgical procedures where something is *done to you*, weight-loss surgery is usually regarded as a collaborative procedure. Your surgeon and the staff know that it's important to keep you informed every step of the way. That's the next level of support you'll receive from your surgeon's office—education. At times, you may feel overloaded with new information. In fact, it's normal to feel the way Jill did: "Oh, the new words I was learning—*bariatric surgery, biliopancreatic diversion*, and others—it was pretty overwhelming!"

Your education will begin with your first office visit. You'll learn about weight-loss surgery and its ramifications. (Having read this book, you'll be familiar with a lot of what you hear.) The surgeon's office will go over the various types of bariatric surgery, the surgeon's procedures, and all of the essential information regarding the specific surgery you choose. You'll also learn about the preoperative protocol and what to expect along the way.

At various points during your journey, you will also probably be speaking with the nurse, program manager, nutritionist, psychotherapist, and a wide range of doctors in other specialties. You will be gaining a comprehensive knowledge of not only the presurgical, surgical, and postsurgical issues but also of your overall health. You are a partner in the process.

You'll most likely receive an information packet or booklet designed by the surgeon's office. This information should help cut through the confusion and anxiety. The packet may include success stories, relevant articles, "what to expect" checklists, and other important information.

With all the changes that are taking place in your body and in your life after surgery, you will continue to need the support of your surgeon's office. It's for this reason that most bariatric surgeons are often referred to as "surgeons for life." This long-term postsurgical support tends to come in three main areas: medical visits, continued education, and help complying with your doctor's orders. Let's take a closer look at the support you'll receive in each of these areas.

Medical Visits

The first area of support is fairly straightforward. For at least the first six weeks after surgery, you will be seen by your surgeon's office on a weekly basis. After that, the frequency of your medical visits will begin to taper off. However, you can be sure they will continue for an extended period of time, perhaps periodically for life. (The frequency of your visits may vary from one physician's office to another. The office staff will inform you how often you will need to return for checkups.)

After surgery, it is extremely important that you keep up with all of your scheduled medical visits. Also, you must notify your surgeon of any problems that arise as quickly as possible rather than wait until your next appointment. To receive the necessary support in this area, it is essential that you keep your surgeon accurately and honestly informed of what is occurring physically and emotionally. It is also very important to be honest about what you've been eating and drinking. However, if you're used to keeping this information to yourself, you may find it difficult to be honest about what you've been taking in to your body. Remind yourself that there's no need for embarrassment. You will not be judged. Accurate reporting of food intake is essential in receiving the medical support you need during this time.

Keep in mind that you've chosen your surgeon because of the trust and confidence you have in his ability. Your surgeon's expertise isn't limited to presurgical examinations and his ability to perform surgery. It also includes his complete understanding of obesity and its comorbidities. We've men-

The Best "Party" in Town

In addition to all the "formal" support you can expect to receive at your surgeon's office, there's often an informal support system in place, which some people fondly refer to as the *waiting-room phenomena* or the *best party in town*. Does this sound strange? In the world of weight-loss surgery, a cheerful, casual atmosphere isn't out of the ordinary. Chances are, the first time you step into the surgeon's waiting room, what will strike you first are the bright, cheerful colors and oversized chairs. (Most of the equipment, you'll discover, is probably oversized as well.) The office staff members will greet you with a friendly smile and a sincere interest in how you are. You've probably spoken to one or more of them on the phone or perhaps you've met them at the support group. If so, they'll probably remember your name. Either way, whether you are familiar to them or not, you will receive a warm welcome.

No matter your size, none of the other people in the waiting room will stare at you. They either are, or were, much like you are. You don't need to fear being judged by them, or by anyone at the surgeon's office for that matter. They all understand where you are coming from.

You may feel a strong sense of belonging and unconditional support from the very beginning, no matter how frightened you were at first. "It was

tioned that during your presurgical exams and even during surgery, it's possible your surgeon will discover that you have a comorbidity. However, even during postsurgical exams, your surgeon or other team member may uncover something that was previously hidden. As you know, hidden comorbidities can be life threatening, so this is just another reason to be sure to keep all of your medical appointments.

Jim tells the following story about an important discovery during one of his postsurgical medical visits: "At my last postsurgical check, a rather startling fact came to light—the nutritionist discovered that I was suffering from adult-onset rickets. It's wonderful that the surgeon has a staff that looks out for us so well. I had been to an orthopedist, a neurologist, a rheumatologist, and a psychologist for the pain, but none of these doctors could figure out what was wrong. However, the team nutritionist picked it up immediately and assured me it could be treated satisfactorily."

You'll probably witness a high level of expertise from each and every member of the weight-loss surgery team, as well as an enormous amount

---

my first visit, and I was scared," said Cindy, thinking back to when she was 310 pounds. "I walked into the waiting room and was surprised by how upbeat everyone was. One of the women waiting to be seen gave another person a beautiful designer dress that no longer fit her. The guy beside me showed me his 'before' picture, and someone else offered me a glass of water. Suddenly, I wasn't quite so scared."

In our waiting room, people often chat comfortably, sharing not only stories of success and failures but also recipes, clothes, vacation shots, and before-and-after pictures. Many of them have developed relationships with one another. Some people are so well liked that others actually try to schedule their office visits around them. For example, our patient John has lost 200 pounds and, at his current weight of 300, he's always quick with a joke to lighten the mood. He feels great about his new weight, and he's continuing to lose. He's an inspiration to others.

You'll likely come across many people like John in the waiting room at your weight-loss surgeon's office. As they share their stories and successes with newcomers and old friends alike, the spirit of support grows. What's more, such people make it evident that there *is* hope and life on the other side. Someday, you may be one of those people who enhance the supportive atmosphere and make others feel at ease.

of compassion and empathy. Often, the rewards of their hard work come in the form of witnessing the continued progress of their patients. At your postsurgical medical visits, the staff will continue to reassure and support you as they did before surgery. In fact, patients often describe the people at their surgeon's office as an extended family or "even better than family."

Continued Education

Before surgery, you did a lot of research and asked many questions to get the information you needed to be fully informed about what you were facing. After surgery, it's just as important to stay informed. Your surgeon's office will provide you with, or direct you to, the information you need to understand the changes your body is going through. You'll find yourself knowing more about your health and your body than you ever thought possible. Not only will you continue to learn about all of the conditions associated with obesity, but you will also stay informed of possible postsurgical complications. The information and support you receive from your surgeon's office will help you take good care of yourself after surgery. For some of you, this self-care has been a long time in coming. This time around, you'll be receiving the medical support you need to properly care for a body you can be proud of.

Help Complying With Your
Weight-Loss-Surgery Program

Your compliance with your weight-loss-surgery program is essential to surgical success and long-term health. After surgery, you will need to comply with all aspects of your program, including keeping your medical appointments (as mentioned earlier), developing new eating patterns, and getting regular exercise. Your surgeon's office will be very helpful in keeping you on track.

Proper food intake is discussed in Chapter 9. Your team nutritionist will probably reinforce much of what you read in that chapter. You're new eating patterns will be far different from what you've experienced in the past. Psychologically, you may have previously regarded food as your best friend. That best friend will be changing. Initially, your intake of food will be greatly curtailed, and weight loss will be rapid. Chances are you'll have little appetite at first. You'll need support in dealing with your rapid weight loss as well as all of the other physical and emotional changes that will be occurring. In later months, you'll need even more support when your appetite and cravings return, sometimes with a vengeance. The surgeon's staff will provide the support you need during these challenges. They'll reassure you that continued compliance with the program is essential, even when it seems most difficult. They may suggest alternative behaviors, sometimes through behavior-modification sessions, and strategies to help you deal with the problem, and will also assure you that this is a normal part of postsurgical recovery.

At some point down the road, you will reach a plateau and stop losing weight, even though you have more to lose. The staff will provide the necessary support and reassurance that this plateau may be temporary. They'll remind you of your success, and that in the interest of long-term health, you must continue to comply with food and diet protocols.

When you were morbidly obese, exercise may have been too difficult for you. However, participating in exercise activities on a regular basis is now very important. The surgeon's staff will stress your compliance with an exercise program and will support you in your exercise endeavors. They'll serve as teacher, friend, cheerleader, and drill sergeant. Be prepared!

FINDING SUPPORT IN YOUR FRIENDS AND FAMILY

If at all possible, your friends and family members need to be essential players in your support network. Unfortunately, as is true for some of our patients, having the support of your family may be a foreign concept to you. There's a chance you may even feel isolated from your closest family members, sometimes because of their unkindness and lack of understanding. For example, Jenny, a 270-pound patient told us, "Growing up, my brother's nickname for me was *fat, ugly dog!* He even wrote those awful words across my picture in the yearbook. I cried when I saw what he'd done and showed it to my parents. My mom told me not to be so sensitive, that it was only a joke, and that nobody else but me would see it. That *joke* hurt me so deeply and made me wonder if I really was a fat, ugly dog."

Tom, at 320 pounds, told us he sometimes felt like an outsider even with his own children. "My youngest daughter—a champion diver on the one-meter board—asked me not to officiate that season because my appearance at the dive meets embarrassed her. My first reaction that spring and summer was to withdraw into myself even deeper—that had become my well-established pattern."

Fortunately, even though some people might feel like outsiders when it comes their closest relatives, this isn't the norm. Most of our patients report that their family and friends provide welcome and wonderful support.

Others have at least a few people who understand them, who they feel special around, and vice versa. Focus on those people in your life. Talk with them earnestly and deeply about your decision to have surgery, as discussed in Chapter 4. Explain which areas you will need help in before and after surgery. Ask them to be honest with you about their willingness to help. If they don't think they can help you, assure them that it's okay to be honest.

Some people may have isolated themselves so much over the years that they think they have no one to turn to. If this is your case, think about someone you may have overlooked or lost contact with. He might be more available than you think. If you feel truly alone, consider attending a local support group on a regular basis. You will likely find people there who have walked in your shoes. They can provide an important source of support.

The following discussions should help you understand what type of assistance you may need from your friends and family.

Presurgical Support

Consider choosing one support person to accompany you to your first weight-loss-surgery support group meeting and your first office visit. At times, you'll be receiving overwhelming amounts of new information, some of which will be technical. It's normal to be nervous and excited during this time, which makes it even more difficult to remember everything you hear. Your support person can serve as an extra ear and a memory aide.

As you become more educated in the range of choices and procedures, your support person can be right beside you in the process. He can assist you in making an informed decision by discussing with you all the details, including the pros and cons.

The decision-making process can be highly emotional due to the risks, commitments, and ultimate gains involved. Your support person can help keep you grounded. He can remind you of the information and options you've heard but may not remember. Also, your support person can help keep you on track and remind you to stay positive. At times, you may request that this person intervene when other family members or friends are reacting to your journey negatively. Your support person can try to help educate these negative people if they are coming from a position of misinformation. If this is not possible, you may request that your support person run gentle interference during the process.

It is not unusual in the weeks before surgery to start having second thoughts. At this point, your support person can help you focus on why you made the decision and why you had concluded that it was right for you. Cassie, for example, struggled hard with her decision to have weight-loss surgery. When she started having second thoughts, she made excellent use of a presurgical support system—her family. "Before I had surgery, it was important to be reminded of all the research I had done and all the careful thought I had put into my decision," she said. "My support system kept me focused. For the two to three weeks before surgery, I was very emotional and had more extreme highs and lows than I'd ever had before. Whenever I fell out of sorts, my family remained calm and grounded. They assured me I wasn't going crazy. They reminded me of all the research I'd done and that my comorbidities were very real and life threatening. They pointed out that I'd chosen an excellent surgeon, and kept me focused on my hopes, dreams, and life on the other side." Although your support person can be very helpful if you're having second thoughts, don't forget that the ultimate decision is yours.

There are practical ways your loved ones can keep you on track presurgically to help ensure surgical success. Later in the book, we'll go into more detail about these practical aspects. For now, it is important to remember that certain presurgical steps—such as being aware of and changing your eating patterns—can enhance optimum long-term postsurgical success. Taking these steps will not be easy, and this is where your support person, as well as your surgeon and nutritionist, will be a great help. Your support person can begin by helping you stock the house with more appropriate foods, by educating your family about the importance of your new eating habits and what they entail, and looking for enjoyable activities that do not center on going out to dinner or cooking up a storm in your kitchen.

It is not unusual for people to go on a large-scale eating binge before starting a new diet. While you may have done this regularly in the past, now is definitely not the time. Your support person will remind you that this "last supper" can create *serious* consequences during surgery.

Because the days preceding the surgery can be very intense, you may find yourself experiencing all sorts of strong emotions. You may be excited, tense, frightened, or anxious. In the past, you may have turned to food to ease your fear or calm your nerves. This time, however, you must depend on your support person to get you through it.

Your support person can also help you begin an exercise routine and, whenever possible, exercise with you. Exercise is key to long-term weight-loss maintenance; presurgically, it strengthens your body for the surgery itself. Your surgeon's office will help you plan the best possible program for you. At this stage, the perfect support person can serve as cheerleader, exercise buddy, and drill sergeant.

Postsurgical Support

The postsurgical period will be a time of great change in all areas of your life on levels you probably would never have expected or even imagined. Relationships, jobs, activities, likes, and dislikes will change. You may look in the mirror and wonder who that person staring back at you is. This can be a frightening and jarring process. During this time, your family and friends can help keep you anchored. Keep in mind also, that postsurgical support can sometimes be a life-or-death issue. Linda's says, "If it hadn't been for my cousin Susan's love and support, I might have died. After surgery, I had some confusing and unexpected complications and a lot was going on. Susan stayed by my side constantly. She kept everything in mind, stayed calm, and kept everyone on point. She was my advocate; my voice and my memory at a time when I felt like I was swimming upstream and could not take responsibility for myself. I know this sounds corny, but it was Susan's love and support that got me through a very tough time."

If postsurgical complications occur in your case, and you find yourself in pain, frightened, and unable to care for yourself, you may need someone like Susan. This person can be your voice at a time when you are not able to explain your problems to the hospital staff. He can seek answers to your questions, let the staff know if something is wrong, and just be your advocate in general to keep the staff "extra interested" in you.

FINDING SUPPORT IN A SUPPORT GROUP

A good support group can offer an invaluable source of compassion, empathy, information, and advice on every aspect of the weight-loss-surgery experience, both physical and emotional. Regularly attending a support group offers the possibility of developing deep and lasting friendships and/or casual acquaintances with whom you simply feel comfortable. Although the groups are primarily for people who have had or are waiting to have weight-loss surgery, anyone can attend. Family and friends are welcome and may quickly become valued members of the group.

Groups may meet weekly, bimonthly, or monthly either at the surgeon's office or in a larger place, such as a hospital or community center. Smaller groups may meet at the home of one of its members. The meetings are generally about an hour long, but others may be as long as two hours or more.

Depending on the particular format of the support group, the leader of the meeting may be the surgeon affiliated with the group, a member of the surgeon's staff, another health professional, or even a postsurgical patient. Regardless of who leads the group, a member of the office staff or the surgeon is usually available at these meetings.

During many support-group meetings, there's time to socialize, for sharing testimonials, and to exchange information. "The support group is a place where we can ask questions of the doctors and patients about what to expect both before and after surgery," said John, who felt confused and alone before attending one of our groups. "Sometimes, we don't know what is 'normal.' We need the encouragement of those who have been there, but also need to hear from those who have failed, even for a short time, so that we can know in advance what to watch out for or avoid."

Some groups plan outings and social events throughout the year, and in some cases, they may even gather together for dinner after a meeting where they can exchange ideas regarding food, nutrition, and eating, preferably with the surgeon in attendance. Some groups even put out a monthly newsletter with notes from the surgeon, staff members, and patients. Not only do such newsletters provide important information, they often also offer heartwarming stories, hope, and humor.

The following sections discuss specific ways your support group can be of help to you at various stages of the process:

Presurgical Support

First and foremost, the support group you attend will be a vital aide in answering the all-important question "Is weight-loss surgery right for me?" At your first meeting, you'll receive a flood of information. You may begin hearing the same information over and over again. That's okay. Repetition is how we learn best. Again, you'll be urged to ask questions. What may strike you the most at your first meeting are the individual patient testimonials. For example:

"My name is Carla. I had my surgery sixteen months ago. I've lost 180 pounds. I have also *lost* my CPAP machine, wheelchair, and walker."

"My name is Mark. I had my surgery eleven months ago, and I've lost 110 pounds. My daughter got married this week, and I walked her down the aisle. It was amazing, and my daughter couldn't stop crying. This time last year none of us expected to see me alive another six months. It's a miracle!"

"My name is Labelle. I had my surgery six months ago, and have lost

80 pounds. I feel great and just look at me! My husband says I'm one hot mama!"

At first, this may seem like a dream come true, so you may not be prepared for what you hear next: "Larry has been readmitted to the hospital once again with complications. Please send him your cards, your e-mails, and your prayers."

In the support group, you will be privy to the good, the bad, and the ugly of weight-loss surgery on a very intimate and personal level. The personal knowledge obtained in the support group is vital in making the best and most-informed decision possible. The support group will help you to realize that you will be giving your informed consent to what is no longer a fantasy, but a serious surgical procedure and a life-changing reality.

Preoperatively, the group will also provide a sense of universality. Most basically, this help has to do with a startling sense of understanding and acceptance. You will enter your first support group tentatively. You will certainly be surprised at the openness and sharing of the longtime group members. You may also be surprised at how happy everyone is to be there. You probably have known for a long time that your weight has ruled every moment and aspect of your life. If you think most people don't understand what it is like to walk in your shoes, the reality is that you are probably right. No matter how much they care about you, no one who has not been there can fully understand what it is like to be morbidly obese. As you listen to the other patient testimonials for the first time in the support group, you will be startled and want to shout, "Hey, that's my story!" For the first time in a long time, you will realize that there are others who feel exactly as you do, who have walked in your shoes, who not only fully and completely understand, but also are willing to talk about what they experience without embarrassment or shame.

As your surgery date approaches, it is normal to feel excited, but also scared. It is normal to be afraid. You may even be having second thoughts about the surgery. You should discuss your fears in the group. Other group members have probably had some of the same fears and can share actions to mitigate the causes of the fears, as well as just listening and validating. You may find that doing something concrete and positive helps alleviate your fears. During this period, group members are the best people to help you move into positive action. Ask them to share tips for healthy living. Their ideas will not only help alleviate fear, make you feel more in control, and give you something concrete to do, but also help you to begin to get your body in the best possible shape to help ensure postsurgical success.

It is common for group members to keep in close personal phone or Internet contact as the day of surgery approaches. You may want one of the group members to accompany you on the day of the surgery itself. This is not an unusual request, and support group members often consider it an honor to accompany a new friend on this significant journey. When you come out of the anesthesia after surgery and return to your hospital room, you may be surprised to find a support group member waiting there. If you have attended the group regularly before surgery, you will likely find many unexpected visitors to your hospital room as well as an onslaught of cards, calls, and e-mails. In many support groups, the postsurgical success of each member is a source of pride for the whole group.

Michael's touching words sum up the important role a support group has in one's life: "When I first joined the weight-loss-surgery support group, I was lost and alone. I needed to find a place where I would be accepted. Not only was I dying emotionally, but I was also close to death because of my morbid obesity. At the time, I just didn't care because everyone in my life had abandoned me. My hope, joy, and self-esteem were gone. I knew I was breathing but wished I would stop. Then, at the support group, I discovered that others had walked in my shoes. They had regained their self-esteem and experienced renewed hope. The warmth and friendliness of the members overwhelmed me, and I began to make new friends almost immediately. Their support, and the support of the whole group, helped me begin to rebuild my life, giving me hope and the power to survive. I know that some of these people will be my friends for life."

Postsurgical Support

After surgery, your support group will continue to be an invaluable source of information. No matter how well you have prepared, you will be surprised by how quickly your body, as well as your mind, is changing. You may be happy with these changes, but the rapid rate at which they happen can be disorienting. The group can help you to deal with all of the myriad and complex aspects of those changes. Your postsurgical keyword will be "different." Nearly everything in your life will be different—your relationships with friends, family, and colleagues; the way people perceive you; your clothing; the activities you participate in; exercise routines; and, of course, the food you eat. Many members of your support group will know exactly how this feels and can provide invaluable tips on how they have weathered those same storms. As time passes, you'll find yourself supporting other members of the group, particularly new members. Not only will you comfort and support others in much the way others supported and comforted you, but you'll also find yourself growing and feeling good about yourself as a result.

FINDING SUPPORT ON THE INTERNET

The Internet is chockfull of informative, reputable websites, chat groups, and message boards that cover nearly every topic imaginable, and that of course includes weight-loss surgery. If you are not Internet savvy, now is a good time to learn how to put the World Wide Web to good use. You'll find many supportive, caring people from all over the country right at your fingertips.

Many weight-loss-surgery programs offer their patients membership in a *listserv*, an Internet communication tool that facilitates the distribution of information. When you are a member of a listserv, you have the opportunity to post questions, comments, or responses to all the members of the group at the same time via your e-mail account. When you submit a posting to the listserv, your submission is distributed to the e-mail inboxes of all the people who subscribe to that list. You do not have to submit postings in order to be a member. You can simply read the posting of others. Here's a sampling of the types of postings you'll likely come across:

I chased my granddaughter down the hall today. I didn't catch her but was hot on her heels! I forgot what it's like to run.

Anyone know a good plastic surgeon in the area?

I got released from the hospital today. I was pretty scared for a while, but I am doing fine now, and appreciated all of your cards, calls, and visits. I loved the dozens of online messages waiting at the house when I got back. I don't know what I would do without you guys. I love you all!

My surgery is scheduled for next week. I am really getting scared. I have a two-year-old. What if I die? Who will take care of her? I guess I know the answer. If I don't have the surgery, I will die for sure. I am so scared. Please keep me in your prayers.

Message boards, also known as discussion boards, are also a great way to communicate with people over the Internet. This is done directly through the website serving the board, rather than via e-mail. You can read messages from other posters and respond to them, or start your own discussion.

What's great about these online support groups is that no matter the time or day, you can sit down at your computer and read or write about your concerns and/or successes. People who have experienced what you're going through—who have been there, or are there, themselves—can provide you with the support or assurances you need during this period in your life. And *you* can be there for them to lend your support. Members may vent their frustration at their insurance companies, ask questions about different surgeons and their weight-loss-surgery programs, share common experiences, and offer advice.

Often, you can get an immediate online response to a critical question you might have, but remember that this advice is informal and doesn't substitute for sound medical advice in an emergency. While other patients' opinions and ideas can be of enormous value, these people are not necessarily doctors or other medical professionals. Therefore, it is essential that you contact your surgeon's office, nutritionist, or psychotherapist if you have medical questions or if you are in medical distress.

Online support groups can supplement your weekly or monthly in-person support groups. Or, if you live in an area where no in-person support group is available, this can serve as your sole support group. Obviously, in this case, the Internet can fill a particularly important gap in your journey.

So, how do you find an online support group? The best place to start is usually with the websites affiliated with your surgeon's office, or ask the surgeon's staff for their recommendations. Sometimes, in-person support groups maintain their own active Internet sites. This additional contact between members can deepen and intensify existing group friendships. So, if your support group has an Internet site, this is also a very good place to start. You can also surf the Internet for other weight-loss-surgery support groups and read the posts on that site for a few days to determine if this group is for you.

Each member of an Internet support group has his own ideas, opinions, and personality. At times, this becomes very apparent and may result in heated arguments or hurt feelings. That's why group postings must be monitored for content. Be sure that the group you belong to has a monitor. Support groups are meant to be positive and supportive. Negative judgment and destructive criticism have no place in these forums. You may already know what it feels like to be excluded, ganged-up on, or diminished. The Web is no place for any of this. The job of the monitor is particularly important to keep things on track and safe!

Chat rooms—discussions that take place in real time—may be another

Sorting Out the Good From the Bad on the Internet

The sheer number of websites devoted to weight-loss surgery makes it difficult to sort out the good from the bad. Which sites provide useful information? Which sites can you rely on? Which sites are misleading or dangerous? Although it sometimes takes an expert to answer these questions, there a few things you can ask yourself that will give you a good idea if a site is reputable or not. For each site you visit, ask the following:

1. Who owns the website? The owner of a website is usually listed on the homepage in the upper-left corner of the screen. A website is likely to be highly reputable if it is operated by well-known organizations such as the American Medical Association or the American Society for Bariatric Surgery; by a university; or by a branch of the U.S. government. (Government sites don't always identify themselves, but you will know a government website if the website address ends in ".gov.") Keep in mind that there are other reputable websites besides those operated by the organizations mentioned. See the Resources section for websites we find particularly helpful.

2. Who is the author of the information on the site? This vital piece of information should be readily available to you on any reputable site you visit. If the author of the information on the site is not disclosed, you will want to look elsewhere for your information.

3. What is the author's background? Carefully consider the qualifications of the author of any information you find on the Internet. Quite often, websites are developed by people who are good at promoting themselves and their wares, but may have little background in the field. Although their credentials may seem impressive, be sure they have degrees you recognize and know are acceptable. Don't be impressed by a string of letters following anyone's name unless you are sure of their qualifications.

4. Does the site seem more interested in selling you something rather than teaching or informing you about a subject? In this case, let the buyer beware. Your surgeon's office should provide you with a list of any helpful products you might need and where you can purchase them. Avoid sites that want to sell you something you probably don't need.

5. How is the website organized? When you visit a site for the first time, take a look at the homepage. Click on items of interest to determine if the site is user-friendly. Unfortunately, some of the very best sources may be poorly organized. There may be so many buttons and/or other options that anyone using it can get lost very easily. Don't waste your time with sites that are difficult to figure out. There are many more to choose from.

6. Does the site make unbelievable claims? Look out for phrases such as "newly discovered," "brand new principle," "revolutionary new drug," "absolutely guaranteed," or other similar, unbelievable claims. If something seems to good to be true, it probably is. Don't waste your time on that site; look elsewhere.

7. Does the site have "hot links"—buttons that take you to other sites? If so, where do those buttons take you? If these links lead you to sites that seem suspicious or fail to disclose important information as mentioned above, the original site itself becomes suspicious. Think about why this site would refer you to, or connect you to, poor-quality sites. We are known by the company we keep, aren't we? The same is true for websites.

Once you've answered all of the above questions, you should be pretty clear on whether or not a website is helpful or if it should be avoided. When visiting various sites, keep in mind that much of the material you find on the Internet is written in an easy-to-understand manner. However, some of the material, though accurate and comprehensive, may be technical and difficult to understand. In these cases, ask a professional for help, if necessary, to more fully understand what've you read before you make any serious decisions or take any action.

source of information and support. They, too, are all over the Internet. However, some of the individuals in chat rooms may not be there to support you. Avoid chatting with people who seem to have some axe to grind, someone "to get even with," a bone to pick, or whose stories seem too incredible to believe. Also, keep in mind that anonymous information can be misleading and possibly harmful.

In any mode of communication with people on the Internet, be sure to consider the points of view of many people rather than simply reading one person's post and taking it as gospel. People's experiences vary—whether they are good or bad. Do a little detective work and look for confirmation from others. Allow for the fact that every treatment, including surgery, has its side effects and complications. Just because someone may have experienced a problem does not mean there is something wrong with the particular treatment or the practitioner. Search for other opinions and do more research before making any conclusions of your own. When dealing with what you read on the Internet, remember that just because something is written down, it doesn't mean it is true. See the inset "Sorting Out the Good From the Bad on the Internet" on page 90.

CONCLUSION

It's clear that having support is essential during this time in your life. If you didn't know where to look for this support, this chapter has shown you all the different avenues you can take to find it. Friends, family, support group members, and your surgeon and his staff can all lend a hand. Remember, you don't have to go through this alone. During this time of your life, your existing relationships have the potential to deepen, you'll make new friends along the way, and you'll find much warmth and empathy from the medical professionals and staff that you'll be dealing with—probably for the rest of your life. Hopefully, you'll also find support in these pages as we continue with you on your journey.

CHAPTER 6

$\mathcal{Y}$OUR FIRST MEDICAL APPOINTMENT AND PRESURGICAL TESTS

The first visit to your weight-loss surgeon's office will probably be unlike any medical visit you've ever had. For most people who select to have weight-loss surgery, visits to a doctor's office for obesity-related health problems are often routine occurrences. These visits may have seemed bothersome at best and degrading or demoralizing at worst.

Having gone to the doctor to feel better, you may have left her office, on more than one occasion, feeling worse—not only physically but emotionally as well. You may have felt that your doctor had limited knowledge of—or, at times, limited compassion for—the issues surrounding obesity. The undersized chairs in the waiting room also might have contributed to your discomfort. Perhaps you noticed other people in the waiting room or even the staff members staring at you. And maybe you stressed over being weighed on the doctor's scale, which only weighs up to 350 pounds, a weight you may have exceeded long ago. Worse yet, you may have made an appointment with your doctor for a condition totally unrelated to obesity, only to be told by the doctor after your exam that you should really consider going on a diet.

Fortunately, your first visit to a weight-loss surgeon's office will be a welcome change of pace. In contrast to other doctor's visits, you are not there to figure out what's wrong with you; you already know. You have a weight problem, and you plan to get the help you need. This chapter will give you some idea of what to expect during your first visit with the surgeon and other specialists. By the time you arrive in your surgeon's office, you will already be a well-informed patient, and you'll know which questions to ask. Hopefully, this chapter will make you feel more comfortable as you go through all the initial steps to eventually reach your goal. Keep in mind that protocol may vary from practice to practice, and your experience may be somewhat different from what's described here. Nevertheless, you'll finish up this chapter with a good understanding of the next steps you will be taking.

SUPPORT COMES FIRST

When you call a weight-loss surgeon's office for the first time, you may expect to be able to make your initial appointment right away, the way you would when calling other doctors. However, in many weight-loss-surgery centers, it is mandatory that you first attend a meeting of a weight-loss-surgery support group affiliated with the surgeon's office unless you are traveling from a long distance. You may be surprised by this and find yourself listing all the reasons you can't make it: *I can't get a babysitter. . . . I live too far away. . . . I have to get up early for work. . . . My book club meets that night. . . . I'm not into groups.* In such practices, the program director, coordinator, or patient consultant will most likely be kind and knowledgeable, but very firm! In response to your excuses, she will probably say something like, "Perhaps this isn't the surgery for you, since you'll need to make many trips here in the next few months." And the next thing you know, you'll find yourself at the support group—and there's a very good chance you'll be glad you went. By that time, you'll probably be impressed by the workings of the whole process.

Janet, a support-group coordinator recalls: "I hated going to the support group that first time. I knew what I wanted in life. When I called the surgeon's office, I was sure I could set up an appointment on Tuesday, have the surgery on Thursday, and begin losing weight by the weekend. I went to the group, sat in the back of the room, and said nothing. I was embarrassed that I'd gotten to the point that I even had to be there. I felt like a failure. Everyone there was warm and friendly, and willing to share to their stories—but not me. They wanted to be my friends. I thought I didn't need any more friends. I was *never* going to get involved—but I'm glad that's not what happened!"

Let's take a look at a typical support group to get a bird's-eye view of the goings-on. This should help familiarize you with what might happen at your support group: Members arrive, mingle a bit, and then take their seats when the meeting is called to order by the group leader. After some general information is dispensed and post-op patients share their testimonials, attendees are often divided into two groups—pre-op and post-op—where they can discuss issues relevant to their stage of the process.

At this point, a guest speaker may give a lecture to the post-op patients on any one of a variety of topics. Occasionally, a member of the group will prepare and give the presentation. A question-and-answer period usually follows a formal presentation.

Meanwhile, pre-op patients and newcomers like you attend a thorough lecture given by one of the surgeons or other experienced staff members affiliated with the center. This lecture covers many of the topics discussed in this book, including a discussion on body mass index. There is usually a brief introduction about obesity and its related health problems. The various types of surgery as well as their pros and cons are explained. This is sometimes accompanied by a slideshow or diagrams and handouts illustrating the procedures. The surgeon speaks briefly about why she has chosen the type(s) of surgery she performs. The final portion of the lecture deals with what to expect after surgery, including possible complications and weight loss. The lecture often ends with a slideshow that illustrates the percentage of improved or "cured" comorbidities in postoperative patients.

Next, the two groups are brought together again and members are given another chance to socialize and ask questions. Over the years, many of the members have not only supported each other but have also become close friends.

If you aren't already aware of the seriousness of the journey on which you are about to embark, you will be after attending a support group. You know that it will not only change your weight and eating habits, but also your life. After attending the support group, you may decide that the surgery is not for you. Chances are, however, that you will be ready to move on to the next step—your first appointment with the surgeon.

YOUR FIRST APPOINTMENT WITH THE SURGEON

After you attend the support group, you'll be able to call the surgeon's office to make an appointment. Having attended the support group, you'll probably have even more questions and concerns. This is good. As mentioned earlier, write your questions down and bring them with you to your appointment. Be sure to bring a copy of the questionnaire in Chapter 4 (see page 60). Also, bring your insurance information and medical-history records.

Consider bringing one of your support people with you to your first visit with the surgeon. This person may have already accompanied you to the support group. The person you choose to bring with you should fully support your decision, or at least respect your decision. Ideally, your support person should have read this book.

The atmosphere of the surgeon's waiting room and the caring concern of the office staff were discussed in Chapter 5. Go back and reread that section to know what to expect when you and your support person step through the door for the first time.

After you've signed in at the front desk, you will most likely be taken into another room to be weighed while your support person waits in the reception area. (You'll probably have to remove only your shoes at this point.) The scale in most weight-loss surgeons' examination rooms can measure up to 800 pounds, sometimes even 1,000 pounds. You may be surprised that you are less embarrassed at the weigh-in than you expected to be. If you weigh more than 350 pounds, it may have been a very long time since you've been weighed since such a scale was previously unavailable to you. David, who weighed 410 pounds at the time of his operation, says, "I went to visit a friend at the hospital. When I left at the end of the day, I passed the loading dock. The workers were leaving for the day, so I waited until no one was in sight. I moved as quickly as I could up on the loading dock and stepped on the cargo scale. I had not been able to see my weight in months. It was humiliating." Like David, many patients have been unable to keep track of their weight after passing the 350-pound mark.

After you've been weighed, you'll either be taken directly to an examination room or back to the reception area. Next, you'll probably be asked to fill out a medical-history form.

Providing Your Medical History

The medical-history form you are asked to fill out will most likely include many of the items you'd find on a standard medical-history form. In addition, you'll be asked to include some or all of the following: a description of why you want the surgery; a list of all of your past and present illnesses, particularly those associated with obesity; your medical history, including hospitalizations, surgeries, and physical or psychological problems; your family's medical history with an emphasis on obese family members and their comorbidities; and a detailed description of previous weight-loss attempts.

The list of comorbidities that apply to you may be extensive. You'll find it very helpful to make a list of these items before your first visit and bring it with you, rather than rely on your memory. Use the list of comorbidities in Chapter 1 to help you put your list together. Don't worry if your list is lengthy. Your weight-loss surgeon will be well acquainted with the vast number of diseases associated with morbid obesity and will not be surprised. Moreover, people with long, detailed lists may have a better chance of receiving insurance coverage for the surgery.

The medical form may question your level of alcohol consumption and smoking habits. Alcohol abuse and smoking increase the risks of the surgery. Most practices require that you stop smoking for six to eight weeks prior to the surgery. Alcohol abuse or excessive alcohol use creates significant problems, particularly in cases of malabsorptive procedures. Therefore, it's extremely important to be honest about your alcohol intake and to seek help if necessary.

Once again, it's a good idea to make a list of all the diets you have tried (including medically supervised diets) along with any relevant information and bring it to your first visit. This list may also be a long one. That's good, since many insurance companies will also factor this information into their decision to provide coverage. The portion of the form concerning your dietary history will ask questions about your fluid intake and what foods you eat, what foods you avoid, how you eat, where you eat, and when you eat. You may also be asked about your current exercise regimen.

Once you've filled out the form, give it to the surgeon or a staff member. The surgeon will likely review the form before you are examined.

Reviewing the Material and Discussing Insurance Issues

After you've been weighed and have filled out the medical-history form, you'll most likely be set up in a small group, sometimes with support members present, to listen to a lecture similar to the one presented at the support group meeting. This lecture is usually given by an experienced staff member.

Although you've already heard much of the information covered in the lecture, it's important to hear it again for a couple of reasons. First, there is a great deal of new information to absorb and think about. Repetition is helpful in this regard. Second, going over the material again reinforces that this is a collaborative effort between the patient and the surgeon and staff. It is essential that new patients fully understand the seriousness of what is about to occur and the permanent lifestyle changes they will need to make in order to maintain their weight loss and return to health.

Generalities about gaining insurance coverage are usually discussed at this time. Any individual insurance issues and problems you may have will be discussed at a later time with a staff member. In any event, be sure to bring all health-insurance-related material to your appointment. (See the section "Insurance Protocol" on page 107.)

Once the lecture is over, you'll be taken into a private examination room. In some cases, you may be able to have your support person present during the exam, but most likely, she will wait in the reception area and rejoin you for your post-examination consultation.

The Medical Examination

Once you're in a private room, you'll probably be asked to change into a gown, which you may be surprised to find fits you quite well. The exam will focus on some of the information contained in the medical-history form and will usually be pretty thorough. Before, during, and after this exam, your questions will be encouraged. You may want to jot some information down on a notepad to help you remember the answers later on. Although you'll be familiar with the risks of the surgery, the surgeon will discuss them with you once again. He'll want to make sure that you are well aware of them and that you still wish to proceed.

Your initial physical exam will be quite thorough, but you'll most likely need to see other specialists and have other tests done before you are cleared for surgery. Therefore, your surgery may still be weeks or months away. In the following sections, we'll take a look at the various specialists you may need to see and the presurgical tests you'll need to have before you're cleared for surgery.

PRESURGICAL TESTS AND CONSULTATIONS

Prior to your surgery, you'll most likely be seeing a wide range of specialists who will be looking for potential problems that must be corrected before surgery for the best possible surgical success. The following tests and consultations—some of which may be performed in your surgeon's office during your initial medical exam or later in a specialist's office—will ensure that you are ready for surgery and will minimize the chance of surprises in the operating room.

Blood Work

Routine blood work is one of the first things that will be required. You'll most likely have blood drawn at your initial visit, but additional tests may be needed. This blood work will include a complete blood count (CBC), a basic metabolic panel (BMP), and a comprehensive metabolic panel (CMP). The BMP is a group of tests that measure salts, sugar levels, and kidney function. The CMP is a group of tests that measure all of the above as well as liver functioning, and fat and protein levels in your blood. The purpose of these tests is to identify problems such as low potassium levels, low protein levels, and abnormal cholesterol levels. ABG (arterial blood gases) testing, which is often required, assesses levels of oxygen in the blood to help determine anesthesia risk. (Consultation with a board-certified anesthesiologist is discussed later in the chapter.) Other blood tests will help to rule out treatable hormone-related problems that may have contributed to your obesity.

Blood tests are also performed to assess nutritional deficiencies. Although it may seem odd, obese people are often malnourished. This can cause not only serious problems before surgery but also even more serious problems after surgery, when lessened absorption contributes to malnutrition. For more information on nutritional status, before and after surgery, see the section "Consultation with a Nutritionist" on page 103.

Abdominal Sonogram

The abdominal sonogram—an image produced by ultrasound—is a simple, non-painful, non-intrusive test that takes about twenty to thirty minutes to perform. While you're lying on the examination table, a technician will run a small hand-held device over the front of your external abdominal area. The test results are almost immediate, but they may not be discussed with you until the surgeon has had a chance to review them.

The purpose of the sonogram is to show the internal appearance of the liver and gallbladder. The abdominal sonogram will reveal the presence of gallstones, which are often seen in the morbidly obese. Gallstones can cause acute inflammation of the gallbladder both before and after surgery. Postsurgical complications are serious, and can lead to fever, pain, and, in extreme cases, blockage of the bile ducts and even gangrene (death of soft tissue) of the gallbladder and jaundice (yellowing of the skin and eyes). Therefore, if gallstones are present, the condition must be treated. In some cases, the gallbladder will be removed during the weight-loss surgery. The procedure is a relatively straightforward one. The bile ducts remain intact after surgery and essentially take over the function of the gallbladder.

Some surgeons do not require this test, particularly if the gallbladder has already been removed.

Echocardiogram (EKG)

Excessive weight often takes a toll on one's heart. These underlying, and sometimes undetected, heart problems can predispose a susceptible individual to sudden cardiac death. Over the years, multiple diets and, some-times, extreme dieting can also stress an already taxed heart. In addition, the use of weight-loss drugs containing phentermine and fenfluramine, often called *fen-phen*, may have caused serious, perhaps undetected, heart problems. (If you have used such drugs—even if it was a long time ago—it is important to notify your surgeon.)

It's important for your surgeon to have knowledge of how your heart is functioning. In many cases, a cardiologist, or heart specialist, will take an electrical recording of the heart, called an *echocardiogram* (EKG), to assess the functioning of your heart and to identify any problems. An echocardio-gram is performed in a similar manner to a sonogram and provides a good picture of the internal structure of the heart.

You may also undergo some stress tests. For example, you may be asked to peddle a stationary bicycle or walk on a treadmill while your heart is monitored to detect any additional abnormalities and to identify limits to your exercise capacity. In some cases, a radionuclear heart test may be nec-essary. This test involves the injection of radioisotopes into a vein. It is generally as safe as a chest x-ray. If indicated, you may need a cardiac catheterization, which involves the insertion of a tube into an artery in your neck or groin that is threaded into your heart. The cardiologist will explain the details. Another possibility is that you will receive an injection of iodine dye through a tube. If you are allergic to iodine, clearly inform the doctor and staff. Be sure you receive a satisfactory response *before* the test begins. All of these tests, including the EKG, are non-intrusive are non-painful. They help identify problems that can be corrected before surgery and help your surgeon to determine the best presurgical and postsurgical treatment for you. They will give you, perhaps for the first time, the clearest picture of your heart's current functioning.

Upper Gastrointestinal Endoscopy or GI Series

An upper gastrointestinal endoscopy is a procedure in which a lighted viewing instrument known as an *endoscope* is inserted through the mouth and down the throat, thereby allowing the surgeon to look at the inner lin-ing of the esophagus, stomach, and the upper part of the small intestine—that is, the upper gastrointestinal tract. This procedure is sometimes called an *esophagogastrodudenoscopy* (EGD). In our practices, upper gastrointestinal endoscopies are routinely done presurgically to identify ulcers, tumors, or acid-reflux-related problems in the esophagus. A tissue sample may be taken to rule out the presence of the bacteria *Helicobacter pylori*. This bacteria is implicated in ulcer disease and certain stomach tumors. If it is present, it must be treated prior to surgery with antibiotics and acid suppressants. Treatment for *Helicobacter pylori* usually requires fourteen days and should be started immediately upon diagnosis.

Many of our patients worry about having this procedure. Although somewhat unpleasant, there is usually little to worry about. First of all, it's performed on an outpatient basis, meaning it does not require an overnight hospital stay. Second, you will be in a "twilight sleep" during the procedure. (Since you will be receiving anesthesia, remember to mention any allergies or difficulties before proceeding. Also, be sure you will have a ride home from your support person.) You shouldn't feel any pain, other than a minor sore throat perhaps, and you will most likely not remember what has occurred.

This procedure is particularly important because it may be the last time a doctor can get a complete look at your stomach to detect any problems. After surgery, a portion of your stomach will be separated off and, therefore, will be inaccessible to the endoscope.

In other practices, surgeons may opt for a GI series instead of an endoscopy. A GI series is an x-ray examination of the esophagus, stomach, and uppermost part of the small intestine. In this procedure, the patient swallows barium sulfate, an opaque substance on x-rays, which outlines the insides of the internal structures quite well. However, a GI series may miss shallow ulcers and small growths, and cannot show any discoloration in the lining of the esophagus, stomach, or small intestine. Moreover, a GI series doesn't provide the opportunity to take a biopsy of the stomach or intestinal lining. Nevertheless, if a person has had previous weight-loss surgery, the upper GI series will help the surgeon determine what's already been done so that she can develop a plan for the upcoming procedure.

Breathing Tests

Many morbidly obese patients suffer from respiratory complications due to upward pressure on the diaphragm or may have other breathing difficulties. Therefore, in our practice, consultation with a pulmonologist, or lung specialist, is mandatory for surgical clearance. She will assess how you breathe and the amount of oxygen you breathe in with each breath. Various pulmonary function tests, as well as a polysomnogram (sleep study; see page 102), help the pulmonologist determine if you are fit for surgery. Chest x-rays, which provide important information about the heart and lungs, are usually taken at this time. Test results from your pulmonologist will help the surgeon and anesthesiologist determine whether or not you will be able to breathe without the assistance of a ventilator after surgery.

If the pulmonologist determines that you are not fit for surgery, you may be required to start and maintain an exercise program for a specified period to increase your lung capacity before the surgery can be performed. In part, this helps prevent postsurgical pneumonia.

During your visit with the pulmonologist, you may also be tested for deep venous thrombosis, dangerous clots that occur in deep-lying veins. There is an increased incidence of this condition in morbidly obese people due to inactivity, edema in the legs, and faulty venous valves in the legs. When present, this condition can bring with it an increased incidence of pulmonary embolism—a clot in the lungs—that can sometimes be fatal. If deep venous thrombosis is indicated, you will require special handling before you can be cleared for surgery.

Sleep Study

A polysomnogram (PSG)—often referred to simply as a *sleep study*—measures your physical state during sleep to identify possible breathing disorders, such as sleep apnea. Sleep patterns, breathing patterns, heart function, muscle activity, brainwaves, and other important factors are all recorded. This painless test takes place in a special facility where you will be required to spend the night. After you've readied yourself for a night's sleep, a technician will attach special diagnostic equipment to various places on your body. The equipment will not cause any pain or discomfort.

If you test positive for sleep apnea, you will need to be treated before you are cleared for surgery. The first line of treatment is the use of a CPAP (continuous positive air pressure) machine, which helps expand the lungs in preparation for surgery. A CPAP titration study, another overnight test, helps determine the proper settings for the machine. Usually, the CPAP machine must before used for at least two weeks before your scheduled surgery. In some cases, a similar machine—a BiPAP (bilevel positive airway pressure) machine—may be used instead of the CPAP. (See page 14 in Chapter 1 for more information on sleep apnea.)

Consultation with the Anesthesiologist

A general anesthesia consultation is always required prior to surgery. Ideally, a board-certified anesthesiologist who works at the hospital where the surgery will take place should do the consultation.

A main concern many of our patients have about the surgery centers on undergoing anesthesia. So be sure to bring any questions or concerns you have to your visit with the anesthesiologist. The answers you receive should reassure you of the safety of the procedure and give you some idea of what actually occurs when you are given anesthesia and what to expect.

Also, be sure your anesthesiologist has received copies of any tests that have been performed, including all the tests mentioned earlier. Also, you'll be asked if you have any allergies and what medications you are currently taking. The anesthesiologist will be especially interested in heart disease or problems, high blood pressure, coronary artery disease, asthma, emphysema, and problems in kidney or liver function. Your airways will be examined to assess potential difficulties with your breathing tube on the day of surgery. You will also be told what to expect on the day of surgery.

Consultation with a Nutritionist

Keeping in mind that many obese people are often malnourished and that proper nutrient intake is very important before and after surgery, it is absolutely essential for pre-operative, as well as a post-operative, patients to consult periodically with a nutritionist. If your surgeon's office does not have a nutritionist on staff, she can usually provide you with a list of experienced nutritionists in your area.

Your nutritionist must be mindful of the metabolic complications involved in surgery for the morbidly obese. Don't be afraid to ask a lot of questions whenever you meet with your nutritionist. This will help her understand your specific needs and areas of concern.

Along with the surgeon, this specialist will review the pre- and post-operative laboratory work to assess your nutritional status. Although this varies from practice to practice, you may be placed on at least two daily supplements presurgically. The nutritionist may review subsequent lab work to make certain that the vitamin, mineral, and protein supplementation is adhered to. She may also use this information to determine whether the intake of certain vitamins or minerals should be increased. The nutritionist will also help you fully understand the lifelong need to take vitamin and mineral supplements. She will stress the likelihood of postsurgical malnutrition without proper supplementation and how it can be a serious problem.

A primary task of the initial visit to the nutritionist is educational—to help you to understand your current eating habits, food choices, and nutrient intake, and to help your nutritionist understand you. You will most likely review your current daily calorie intake, including the source of these calories. This can be used as a baseline for setting up your diet program as well as for comparing levels after surgery. It can also help you more clearly understand problem areas that may be a source of difficulty after surgery. Be sure to be upfront about your current eating habits, including emotionally triggered eating and your favorite problem foods.

In preparation for your initial consultation with the nutritionist, keep a list of *everything* you drink and eat (large portions as well as nibbles) during the course of a day, for at least three days prior to the visit. The list can simply include the time of day and what you ate, or you can make it as involved as you like. Don't rely on your memory; it's usually very difficult to remember everything you've eaten, especially with so much going on. Have your list handy so you can refer to it during the meeting. Also, bring along a list of *all* supplements and medications you are currently taking, including over-the-counter medications such as aspirin. Remember to include any herbal and homeopathic remedies. (It's a good idea to keep a copy of this list in your wallet and update it as needed for future reference.)

The nutritionist will likely put together an eating program for you, tailored specifically to your needs. You'll probably begin to focus on your new eating program from day one, which will likely require a decrease in carbohydrate consumption and an increase in protein consumption. You'll also learn about proper fluid intake and the importance of staying properly hydrated.

In our practice, we stress the importance of beginning your future eating program presurgically to not only lose weight and increase surgical safety, but also to get you into the habit of your new eating patterns. Many doctors believe that the presurgical eating compliance is a sign of dedication to the new program, an awareness that the surgery is not a quick fix, and a good indicator of postsurgical success.

The nutritionist—as well as the mental-health specialist (discussed below)—will also be assessing your food habits for possible eating disorders, including anorexia, bulimia, binge-eating disorder, compulsive overeating, and night-eating syndrome, as well as laxative and diuretic abuse. These disorders can cause serious postsurgical medical complications and must be successfully dealt with prior to surgery. Some people try to hide eating disorders from the specialists in fear of being refused for the surgery. Don't do this! This denial can have deadly consequences! Be honest with your nutritionist and mental-health specialist about any eating disorders you might have. They will assist you in finding help to get the eating disorder controlled before the surgery takes place. Honesty and appropriate action are crucial!

Food tolerances and preferences vary widely from person to person. Postsurgically, the nutritionist will help monitor and adjust your foods and supplements for the best possible long-term result.

Consultation with a Mental–Health Specialist

A mental-health evaluation is often a requirement for insurance coverage as well as for surgical clearance by your surgeon. Both your insurance company and surgeon want to know that you completely understand the procedure and that you are looking at it realistically, from a trained therapist's point of view. Your surgeon's office will most likely give you a list of qualified therapists to choose from, or you may see someone closely affiliated with the practice right in the surgeon's office.

Rather than a talk-therapy session, the mental-health professional you see at this time will be performing a diagnostic evaluation and will ask you a series of questions. Whenever possible, be sure that the person evaluating you is well versed not only in the surgical procedure itself but also on all aspects of what it is like to be morbidly obese. Speaking with someone who really understands your issues can make this more than just a diagnostic tool. Morbid obesity often makes for a pretty rocky road, and you may never have had the chance to talk about what your life has really been like with a knowledgeable professional or otherwise. If you are able to speak freely, you may be able to resolve some of the old pain, while new aspects of your life may be opened up and the road to long-term health will be made clearer. Don't be afraid to ask questions.

Many of our patients worry that they will be turned down for insurance coverage or for the surgery itself as a result of the mental-health evaluation. Although this isn't unheard of, it is rarely the case, although the mental-health practitioner may suggest additional treatment. Surprisingly, after the evaluation, many of our patients discover that they wish to continue talking to the evaluator or other mental-health specialist on a more regular basis.

Being familiar with what you may be asked during the evaluation can be helpful. In all evaluations, you will be asked about your knowledge of the surgical procedure. Don't worry: you aren't expected to know complicated medical information. What the evaluator will be looking for is that you have a general knowledge of the procedure and the potential benefits and risks, including the risk of death. She will want to see that you have an understanding of the necessary postsurgical changes in your diet and that you understand the risks of noncompliance with these dietary changes and other lifestyle changes.

You'll probably be asked why you want the surgery. You might want to write this out and review it before the evaluation so you can clearly communicate all of your reasons for wanting the surgery. Don't forget to mention any comorbidity you have, as well as quality-of-life issues—that is, how your weight has impeded your relationships, your activity level, and even your ability to do ordinary things. You may also be asked what you expect from the surgery and how you feel about the possibility that you will not lose all of the desired weight. The therapist will also probably want to know about your commitment to eating less and changing your lifestyle. She may also ask about your willingness and ability to get adequate and complete follow-up care.

During the course of the evaluation, which may consist of one or two sessions, the evaluator will be taking notes for her report, which will include a brief synopsis of your life, your weight history, and your dieting efforts. She will also take note of your eating behaviors and patterns. Your family history relating to health and weight will also be taken. This aspect of the evaluation looks for the genetic and environmental factors in weight and physical and mental health.

In some cases, you may be asked to take written tests, such as the Beck Depression Inventory, the Three Factor Eating Questionnaire, the Weight and Lifestyle Inventory, or a host of other paper-and-pencil tests. This is not a cause for alarm. It does not necessarily mean you have more serious issues. It may be the manner in which that particular evaluator operates.

Part of the evaluator's report will include a brief mental-health status report with her diagnostic impressions. In all cases, the evaluator will be doing a simple risk assessment. She will want to determine if you have the capacity to give informed consent; whether there is a postsurgical risk of serious psychological complications; and the likelihood of your failure to comply with the program, which may result in serious weight regain or medical complications.

The evaluator will probably also want to know about family cohesiveness and relationships. This is important to be sure that you have the all-important support network available postsurgically as your body begins to heal and you go through emotional changes. If your family members are not able to provide support, let the evaluator know what other arrangements you have made or plan to make.

Aside from reviewing your notes about your reasons for having the surgery, you don't need to "prepare" for the mental-health evaluation—relax. A good evaluator will ask you many questions and will be easy to talk to.

Be as honest as possible. Keep in mind that mental-health evaluations rarely exclude people from having the surgery. What you may discover, is that, like so many of our patients, you'd like to go back and talk some more!

INSURANCE PROTOCOL

Once a surgeon has accepted you as a candidate for weight-loss surgery, she will send a "Letter of Medical Necessity" to your health-insurance company. You may also need to provide your insurance company with a letter from you explaining your need for the surgery in your own words. (See the inset "To Whom It May Concern" below.)

If, after reviewing the information, the insurance company agrees to cover you, it will send your surgeon's office a "Predetermination Benefits Letter." This letter usually states that the weight-loss surgery is "a potential covered benefit." Thereafter, the surgeon may forward a copy of this letter to the hospital where the surgery will take place, together with the contact information of your health insurer's pre-certification company. Someone from the hospital will contact the company to confirm your coverage.

To Whom It May Concern

At some point early on in the process of qualifying for surgery and insurance coverage, you will probably be asked to write a letter explaining your need for weight-loss surgery, primarily for the purposes of obtaining insurance coverage. It's essential that you be your own best supporter in presenting the strongest possible case in favor of weight-loss surgery. The letter should include a description of your obesity-related problems, including quality-of-life issues, as well as a list of your innumerable diet attempts and failures.

If you have difficulty drafting this letter, ask your surgeon's office or members of your support group who successfully got coverage to share their letters with you. To help you on your way, take a look at this outstanding letter written by one of our patients, Patricia Bauer (not her real name).

To whom it may concern:

My name is Patricia Bauer. I am a thirty-five-year-old morbidly obese woman. I am writing this letter in order to obtain approval for weight-loss surgery.

I am 5 feet 4 inches tall. My ideal weight is between 125 and 142 pounds. I currently weigh 349 pounds. My highest weight was 512 pounds. As a result of my obesity, I have developed many health problems, which have kept me from being able to work and therefore caused me to go on Social Security disability income.

Within the past five years, I have been diagnosed with several comorbidities. I have type-2 (non-insulin-dependent) diabetes. I have to check my blood sugar every day and take two types of oral antidiabetics daily. Cuts and bruises take forever to heal. I'm always either thirsty all day, or I'm having to urinate frequently. I often develop highly resistant vaginal yeast infections due to my diabetes. In 1998, I developed a Bartholin's cyst due to my diabetes, which was also resistant to antibiotics and required surgery. I am told that it can recur.

I have severe sleep apnea and must use a CPAP machine at a setting of 12. I have been on the CPAP for over a year and still go to sleep worrying about whether or not I might just completely stop breathing altogether while I sleep.

I also have profound hypersomnolence due to the amount of weight I must carry around. I fall asleep very easily in the middle of the day. This puts me at risk of falling asleep while driving or while cooking. I have to take Ritalin four times a day to combat this.

My weight has caused problems with my back, neck, feet, and knees. I am almost always in pain. I cannot go to certain places because of the far walk from the parking lot. I have handicapped parking permits. I've had to buy orthotics for my shoes just to be able to walk short distances. Oftentimes, when I walk around my apartment barefoot, I get cramps in my feet. This joint pain has caused me to miss a lot of family events such as weddings and birthdays, because I can't get around easily. Life is happening all around me, and I can't participate in it.

I have high cholesterol that has gone as high as 450. This, of course, has put me at great risk of having a heart attack and/or a stroke. I also have urinary stress incontinence. This is not only embarrassing but also causes an irritation that takes days to get rid of. This is particularly worrisome when allergy season comes around. I start sneezing a lot, which causes my stress incontinence to act up.

I've been treated for depression for twelve years. My therapist and psychiatrist agree that my weight issues are my main mental-health concerns. My weight has caused great emotional pain and clinical depression.

I've experienced job discrimination and devastating ridicule by strangers. I try to avoid this kind of pain by not going out in public. Losing this weight would help me improve my self-esteem by providing a more positive self-image and thereby decreasing my depression.

My family's medical history includes morbid obesity on both sides. My mother has type-2 diabetes, and had a heart attack and cardiac bypass surgery. She also has angina. My father had a heart attack seven years ago along with a triple cardiac bypass. He also had type-2 diabetes and hypertension. A few months ago, he suffered a second heart attack, and, recently, passed away in my arms. I am at risk for these ailments as well.

I began my twenty-year battle against morbid obesity when I was fifteen. That is when I began my first doctor-supervised diet program. Since then I have been on Optifast, NutriSystem, and several reduced-calorie diets (all doctor supervised). I've been on Tenuate, fen-phen, Pro-Phen, and plain phentermine. I've seen psychiatrists, therapists, and even went to an eating-disorders program. I've tried several non-doctor-supervised diet programs as well. I've been to Weight Watchers, Overeaters Anonymous, Food Addicts Anonymous, Sugar Busters, Atkins, and prayer meetings. None of these diet and exercise programs worked in the long run. Soon after the initial weight loss, I would gain back all the weight that I lost and then some.

I feel that this surgery is my last hope at alleviating some of my life-threatening health conditions. This is a rather drastic step to take, and I do so with a lot of thought and preparation. I've been going to support-group meetings for the last eight months. I've done a lot of research on this subject. This surgery is supported by a great number of institutions.

I know this surgery is not a quick fix for all my health problems. I know that I will be under a doctor's care for the rest of my life. I know there will be food restrictions as well as nutritional guidelines and an exercise program that I will have to follow. I will continue to participate in the weight-loss-surgery support group. This is not a magical cure. It is, however, a tool that works when used properly.

I have some simple goals. I would like to choose restaurants based on the food, not on whether I will be able to fit in the seats. I want to ride in a car with a seat belt that can be buckled. I want to be able to sit in a coach seat on an airplane. I want to be able to bend over to tie my shoes without running out of breath. I want to walk to the mailbox without pain. I want to be able to walk up stairs without having to gasp for air.

But mostly, I want to be able to do two things: Finish my education, get a job, and get off of disability and out of Section 8 public housing (I have already returned to school and am doing extremely well with a 3.73 GPA) and to not cut my life short due to morbid obesity.

Thank you in advance for your consideration.

Sincerely yours,

Patricia Bauer

CONCLUSION

In this chapter, you learned about what to expect at your first medical appointment with your surgeon. It's true that your experience may be a little different from what's described here, but at least you'll have some idea of what's to come. You also have some idea of what presurgical tests are required and which specialists you may have to see. The importance of consulting with a nutritionist as well as a mental-health specialist should be clear after reading this chapter.

There's so much to do in the weeks before surgery that the actual day of surgery may arrive quite suddenly. The next chapter will give you some idea of what to expect in the days before and the day of your surgery.

CHAPTER 7

*T*HE DAYS BEFORE
AND THE DAY
OF SURGERY

You've gone through all the necessary tests and exams, and your surgeon has become aware of and has addressed any health conditions that may interfere with a successful outcome. Finally, your surgeon and other specialists have cleared you for surgery. You've also received pre-approval for the surgery from your health-insurance company. It's probably been a long time coming, but the day of your surgery is drawing closer. In this chapter, we'll take a look at how to prepare for your stay in the hospital and when you return home, what generally happens the few days before surgery, and what you can expect on the day of your surgery.

You'll certainly have a lot on your mind at this time, so it helps to start making preparations and becoming familiar with this information even before you receive a scheduled date for the procedure. Then, once you receive your surgery date, you can review the material in this chapter again. This should help eliminate any surprises or forgotten items.

PRESURGICAL PREPARATIONS

Now that you have a date for your surgery, you are beginning your final countdown. You need to make sure that you have all the bases covered. To help in your preparations, the following sections describe those things you will need to take care of prior to undergoing surgery. A handy checklist follows these discussions.

Verify Approval for Extended Sick Leave From Work

By this time you should have already received approval from your employer for time away from the office for at least four weeks following laparoscopic surgery or six weeks following open surgery. Be sure that you have been scheduled for the maximum amount of time, because it may be difficult to extend your sick leave if necessary. If you can go back to work sooner than expected because you are feeling well, that's great, but don't schedule less time than you may need for recovery.

Review the dates of your time off with your boss to make sure you're both on the same page. Confirm any arrangements you've made with other coworkers or temps who will be handling your workload.

Verify Arrangements for Blood Donors

Blood transfusions are necessary in only a small percentage of weight-loss-surgery cases. However, you may want the hospital to have a supply of blood on hand from people you know and trust (who share your blood type) in the unlikely event you need a transfusion. It is your responsibility—or the responsibility of a designated support person—to make all arrangements with the blood bank. Your surgeon's office should be able to tell you how to go about doing this if you should elect to do so.

Those willing to donate blood to you will need to contact the blood bank at least three days prior to the day of surgery. This is mandatory in order to allow time for laboratory testing and shipment of the donated blood. The donors will also need to sign the necessary papers to make sure their blood is designated for you in the event you need it. (If you do not need the blood during your hospitalization, it will be released for use by other patients.) Contact the blood bank well beforehand to check on the proper protocol.

Keep in mind that donors can be turned down for a number of reasons, such as low iron levels or poor veins, so you'll want to have a few willing donors. If a direct donor's blood type is not compatible with yours, don't worry, the blood bank can still take his donation and provide you credit for a unit of blood that you may receive if needed. In some cases, you may be able to donate your own blood, although this can be expensive. Again, check with the hospital if this is something you may be interested in doing.

Review Which Medicines to Take Before and After Surgery

At least a few weeks before your surgery, your surgeon will inform you which medications you should be taking before and after surgery. You should already be familiar with this information, but review it again with your surgeon one last time at least a few days before the surgery.

Be sure to discuss *all* medications and supplements you are taking, prescription *and* over the counter. This information is very important. For example, many common over-the-counter medications and supplements such as *Ginkgo biloba* can affect blood clotting and result in excessive bleeding following surgery. As your surgeon will already have told you, any substance that affects blood clotting must be discontinued at least two weeks prior to surgery. Also, some other medication must be discontinued. For example, the diabetes medication Glucophage must be discontinued seventy-two hours prior to surgery to prevent serious complications. Make sure you fully understand your surgeon's orders concerning the medication and supplements you should or should not be taking.

It's important to be honest about any and all pills you are taking—even if you realize you shouldn't have been taking it—since keeping this information a secret can have dire consequences.

Stock Up on Postsurgery Medication and Supplements

Make a list of the surgeon-approved medications for use following surgery, and stock up on a month's supply of them, at least a few days prior to your surgery. Don't wait until you are discharged from the hospital to fill prescriptions for painkillers and any other medication you may need. Instead, ask your surgeon to provide you with these prescriptions in advance. If you are already in the hospital, give the prescriptions to a support person who can fill them for you before you return home.

If you are going to be staying at a friend's house or in a nearby hotel following surgery, pack a bag of all of the approved postsurgical medications and bring the bag with you to the hospital. These medications will remain in the bag while you are in the hospital. Hospital rules forbid you to take medication that you bring from home while you are admitted as a patient. Any medications you need during your hospital stay must be supplied by the hospital staff.

Also stock up a month's supply of any required postsurgical supplements, such as chewable multivitamins, calcium supplements, and protein shakes or mixes. You were probably given a list of the items you'll need, but if you do not know which supplements are required, be sure to ask your surgeon or nutritionist in advance so you can have these items on hand when you are discharged from the hospital.

Make Arrangements for Postsurgery Meals

For the first two or so weeks following your surgery, you'll most likely find it very difficult to go food shopping. Therefore, you'll want to shop for the recommended food supplies in advance so you'll have them in easy reach during your recovery period. Shop for a two-week supply of food and liquids. If you aren't sure what you'll need, ask your nutritionist to provide you with a list.

Find a support person who is willing to shop for you when you run low on food during your recovery period. If no one is available to do your shopping, keep in mind that some grocery stores may deliver for a small additional fee. You may want to call a few grocery stores in your area ahead of time to see if this option is available to you.

For some helpful tips on postsurgery food preparation, see the inset "Preparing and Storing Puréed Food" below.

Preparing and Storing Puréed Food

For the first four to ten weeks following surgery, you will be permitted to eat only puréed foods. (The exact amount of time you'll need to eat this way varies with the type of surgery you've had and with the surgeon's preferences.) Baby food is always an option, but some people simply don't like it. Fortunately, you can prepare your own tasty puréed meals using the foods approved by your nutritionist.

You'll need to have a blender or food processor on hand for meal preparation. Cook your food as you normally would. Allow it to cool somewhat before processing. Add any approved herbs or spices for flavor. Set the blender or food processor on purée and run until the mixture reaches a smooth consistency.

You'll probably want to purée different foods separately, but don't be afraid to try different combinations if you think that might suit your taste buds. (Speaking of taste buds, be aware that weight-loss surgery often changes one's sense of taste, so don't be surprised if you discover that you have different likes and dislikes after your surgery.)

Chances are you'll wind up with more puréed food than you can eat at one sitting, so store the extra in freezable containers or bags in one-serving portions in the freezer. (An ice-cube tray is also an option, but be sure to cover it with plastic wrap.) Label the containers with special freezer-compatible pens or labels so you know what's inside.

When you're ready for your next meal, simply defrost your choices in the microwave or on the stovetop. This way, you'll be able to make your own meals in no time at all and with very little effort!

Purchase a Pill Crusher and a Thermometer

Your surgeon will probably advise you to crush all non-liquid medications and mix it with liquid or puréed food for a month or so following surgery. This will prevent pills or capsules from getting "hung up" in your stomach pouch where they could irritate the pouch lining or partially block the outlet. Most drugstores carry pill crushers, so it should be pretty easy to find one. Some pharmacists can liquefy your medications for you; ask your surgeon if this is an option for any of the medications he prescribes.

While you're at the drugstore picking up your pill crusher, also purchase a good thermometer. After surgery, you'll want to monitor your temperature daily or anytime you feel unusually warm or have the chills, since a fever can be an early sign of problems following your surgery. If your temperature is 101°F or higher, contact your surgeon's office.

Arrange for a Suitable Place to Sleep

Make sure that you have a suitable bed or a nice, wide, comfortable recliner to sleep in after surgery. (By the way, waterbeds are not suitable because they are difficult to get out of.) If your bedroom is on the second story, you might want to set up temporary sleeping quarters on the first floor so you do not have to worry about climbing stairs. In certain cases, your surgeon may approve temporary use of a hospital bed to be covered by your health insurance. If you're interested in this possibility, speak to your surgeon and your health-insurance representative.

Make Sure to Have Loose-Fitting Clothing on Hand

Tight-fitting clothing can irritate the site of your surgical incision. This can cause inflammation and "set up" the area for infection. To reduce the risk of infection, wear loose-fitting clothing and bedclothes that are a size or two *larger* than the size you normally wear. Avoid anything with an elastic waistband, including undergarments, for the first few weeks after surgery.

Confirm Your Arrangements for Child Care and Pet Care

If you have small children, you'll need to make arrangements for their full-time care while you're in the hospital and for at least one to two weeks during your recovery at home. You may have friends or relatives who have agreed to take on this responsibility or you may have decided to hire a temporary qualified housekeeper/nanny. Confirm your arrangements with whomever will be watching your children. You may wish to have a backup in the event unexpected circumstances interfere with the first person's commitment to care for your family.

You'll also need to make arrangements for any pets you might have. If your friends or family are unavailable for this task, you can consider boarding your pet at the vet's office while you're in the hospital (keeping in mind you'll have to make arrangements to have your pet returned to you). You might also consider hiring a pet-sitter to come to your home a few times each day to provide for your pet's needs.

Place Your Mail and Newspapers on Hold

If you live alone, contact your local post office and place your mail on hold

---

Get Ready to Track Your Progress

While you're at the drugstore picking up your pill crusher, thermometer, and any other supplies you might need, stop by the stationery aisle and pick out a decorative notebook or two to be used for tracking your postsurgical progress. This is a fun way to document the changes you're about to face.

Many weight-loss-surgery patients who have lost massive amounts of weight naturally want to exercise their "bragging rights" about "how big they used to be." With such a journal in hand, this is easy to do. You can start by pasting current pictures of yourself (front view and side view) on the first page along with the date. Below these pictures, record your weight and waist, hips, and thigh measurements and any comments. Do this periodically—perhaps every month or two—until you reach your goal. Keep in mind that even when you reach a so-called plateau, looking back at what you once weighed and how you looked will give you needed encouragement. In addition, you'll most likely still see your measurements shrinking so it helps to write them down even after you stop losing pounds.

Perhaps you've avoided having your picture taken in the past and don't want to have one taken now. That's fine; just record your weight and measurements. Keep in mind, however that many postsurgery patients are disappointed that they did not have any "before" pictures taken to remind themselves or prove to disbelievers just what condition they were in before surgery. (A driver's license photo shows only so much.) So, to allow yourself those good-hearted "bragging rights" after your dramatic weight loss, go ahead and get your picture taken at least once before surgery.

for the time you'll be at the hospital so it doesn't pile up in your mailbox. Do the same with any newspapers you regularly receive. (A stuffed mailbox and a pile of newspapers on your doorstep are surefire indications that you're away.) Alternatively, arrange for a willing neighbor or family member to take in your mail and papers each day.

Plan for the Payment of Bills

If you are the bill-payer in the family, you'll want to make sure your bills get paid on time while you're in the hospital. Since most household expenses are recurring, you can prepare a pile of postdated checks to be sent out on specified dates. If you are Internet savvy, you can set up an electronic system in which your bills are automatically paid on specified due dates.

Do Your Housekeeping

A few days before you check into the hospital, thoroughly clean your home, including washing, drying, and folding your laundry. It's wise to leave your house or apartment in good order, and when you return home you'll be glad you did. You will probably find that you are too tired to do this type of housekeeping in the first few weeks while you're recovering from your surgery. You may want to ask a friend or relative, or hire someone, to do some light housekeeping periodically until your energy level improves and you feel well enough to do it for yourself.

Make Sure Everything's Runny Smoothly

It's a good idea to make sure that all of your appliances, and especially the family car, are in good working order. Bring your car in for a tune-up a few weeks before the scheduled surgery to make sure that nothing will go wrong if the car is needed for an emergency. Also, be sure you have enough gas in the gas tank. Make certain that essential appliances like your blender, food processor, refrigerator, and stove are all functioning properly. You'll be relying on them after the surgery and wouldn't want them to break down just when you need them.

Update Your Will and Prepare a Living Will

An updated last will and testament and a living will are two very important legal documents to have on hand at all times, not just when you're facing surgery. A last will and testament tells the courts and your family who should handle your estate and how your assets and possessions should be distributed in the event of your death. A living will is a document that clearly expresses your wishes concerning the use of artificial life-support systems and usually appoints someone to make important health-care decisions on your behalf in the event you are unable to do so for yourself. An attorney or legal service can prepare these documents for you. Alternatively, there are standardized forms available in many states, and you can simply fill in the blanks; ask your surgeon's office or the hospital if they have any of these forms.

Confirm Your Arrangements for Company in the Hospital and at Home

It's wise to arrange for someone to be with you in your hospital room after your surgery such as your spouse, friend, older child, religious group member, or support group member. Such a person can help you with basic tasks when you cannot easily help yourself. There may be times when you need help, sometimes quickly, but are unable to get a nurse to come to your room. Your support person may be able to help you or, at least, will be able to go to the nursing station or nursing supervisor's office, if necessary, to get someone to help.

You'll also want to have someone help take care of you for a week or so following surgery. Perhaps a few support people can take turns helping you out, or maybe you have one person who is willing to stay with you. (Help at home with childcare, household tasks, and shopping is an extra bonus.)

If you don't have anyone to help you while you're recovering, discuss this with your surgeon and ask for a week or so in a rehabilitation center if feasible. If yours is an unusual case, particularly if you've experienced complications, your surgeon may agree that you are a good candidate for rehab and will write an order for it in your hospital chart. The appropriate hospital coordinator will seek insurance approval and, if this is granted, will make arrangements for your transfer into such a facility at the time of your hospital discharge. In certain instances, this arrangement can be made prior to your hospital admission.

Confirm Hotel Reservations, If Any

If your surgeon's office is two or more hours away, you may find it helpful to stay in a hotel—accompanied by your support person—for one to two weeks after you're discharged from the hospital. Speak with your surgeon about this possibility. This will help you avoid making a long trip to the office for postsurgery follow-up as well as for any simple problems that might arise. (Be aware that during the first couple of weeks, an otherwise simple problem may become complex if you are hours away from your surgeon's office.)

Don't wait until the last minute to make your hotel reservations. Make them well in advance and call to confirm a few days prior to your surgery. Don't forget to check with your surgeon's offices for advice on local hotels and any possible discounts.

Practice Coughing, Deep-Breathing, and Leg-Pumping Exercises

Two of the more common serious problems following weight-loss surgery are lung conditions such as pneumonia and blood clots that can form in the deep veins in your legs called *venous thrombosis.*

You can help prevent pneumonia postsurgically by practicing coughing and deep breathing for at least a few days before you are admitted to the hospital. Since breathing into your abdomen will be somewhat painful for at least a couple of weeks following surgery, you'll need to use your chest muscles as much as possible. Place your hands lightly across your chest, and breathe deeply. Feel your lungs and chest expanding with the inhalation. Once you've taken as deep a breath as you can, exhale until your lungs are empty. Take ten breaths this way. Perform this exercise several times a day; after each session, practice coughing a few times as well. After surgery, you'll need to do deep-breathing exercises using an apparatus called an *incentive spirometer,* every waking hour to prevent pneumonia. (In fact, your surgeon will likely give you an incentive spirometer to practice with well before your surgery date.) By exercising your lungs in this manner, you'll be much less likely to develop pneumonia or a condition called *atelectasis,* which can cause a fever following surgery.

To help prevent the formation of blood clots, particularly in your lower extremities and pelvis, you'll need to encourage good blood flow in your veins by doing leg-pumping exercises. Performing these exercises regularly helps keep platelets, the factors in the blood that cause clotting, from clumping together and developing into a blood clot.

To perform the leg-pumping exercises, sit or lie down on your back with your legs extended in front of you. Flex your feet backward and forward as far as possible to stretch your calf muscles to their maximum. Do this a dozen or so times several times over the course of the day. After surgery, you'll need to do your leg-pumping exercises every waking hour.

Be sure to practice all of these exercises frequently prior to surgery so that they become second nature. After surgery, it is imperative that you perform these exercises regularly to reduce the risk of developing serious complications.

Work on a Useful Technique for Getting Out of Bed

For a week or more following your surgery, you'll have some difficulty getting up from a lying position. Therefore, you'll want to work on a useful technique to get out of bed. While lying in bed, imagine that you've already had your surgery. Roll over onto your side to the nearest edge of your mattress. Keep your elbow on the mattress, supporting your upper body. At the same time, slide your feet and legs across the bed until they dangle over the edge of the mattress. Then, let gravity bring your legs and feet toward the floor, push your upper body away from the mattress with your elbow and arm. Try this maneuver again and again until you get the hang of it.

Learn to Think Positively

It's normal to feel nervous before surgery, but if you can't relax at all—that is, if you're overly anxious—you'll want to practice positive thinking, also called *positive imagery*. Many people find this technique very soothing during the days leading to surgery.

To practice positive imagery, think of all the wonderful goals you will accomplish with your massive weight loss and see them in your mind's eye as if they've already occurred. For example, picture yourself at a clothing store buying clothes right off the rack. Or see yourself sliding into a small car and fitting comfortably behind the wheel. Or perhaps picture yourself getting that raise or promotion you've always wanted. You can imagine any number of wonderful things you will eventually accomplish.

Jot down all of these positive thoughts on a piece of paper or in your journal. Make a copy for your wallet so you can look at it each time you have any doubts about proceeding with the surgery. Once again, see all of those good things you are looking forward to as if they've already happened.

Pack Your Bags for Your Hospital Stay

To avoid rushing around just before leaving for the hospital, pack your bags a few days before you are scheduled to go. You'll want to bring items of necessity such as your toothbrush, toothpaste, hairbrush, and shaving gear, as well as other items such as hairspray and makeup. Although most hospitals provide disposable slippers, you may feel more comfortable wearing your own. Likewise, you will probably want to bring along other comfort items such as your own pajamas, a special pillow, a pillow cover, or a "cough pillow"—a firm pillow that you can press over your abdomen to help reduce pain when you cough. Don't forget to pack the loose-fitting clothing mentioned earlier. Avoid bringing anything of value, such as jewelry, with you to the hospital since you will probably not have a secure place in which to store them while you're sleeping or when your room is unattended. Have a small amount of money on hand to cover expenses such as a daily newspaper, but keep it in a safe hiding place. We also advise bringing a package of cornstarch with you. Sprinkling a couple tablespoons of cornstarch on your sheets each day will help your body slide around more comfortably and will keep you from "sticking" to the sheets when you perspire. Doing this is perfectly acceptable, and you do not need permission from the hospital staff.

YOUR LAST "NORMAL" MEAL

You are well aware that your eating style will be much different after surgery. As surgery approaches, you've likely thought about this change quite a bit. Food may always have been a source of comfort for you like a good old friend who's always been there for you. It's normal to be concerned about losing the ability to eat all you want, whenever you want, so perhaps this has been a nagging concern of yours.

For one to two days before surgery, you will be placed on a liquids-only diet. Before starting the liquids-only phase, some people are tempted to have one last big meal, which many patients jokingly call "the last supper." This is quite understandable, but every now and then, it can cause serious problems, especially when every meal prior to surgery becomes the last meal. For example, our patient Emma had her "last supper" at every meal for three months after she'd been accepted for surgery. The day before surgery, Emma weighed twenty-five pounds more than she had at her last visit; she'd also become very short of breath just getting up onto the exam table. We had no choice but to cancel her surgery and instruct her to lose this additional weight before we would reschedule the surgery. Unfortunately, Emma didn't cooperate and never returned for the surgery. Since then, she's been hospitalized at least twice for heart and lung problems.

So, let's get real about what you are after here—is the gorging of large quantities of food the way Emma did something you really want to keep as

Checklist for Presurgical Preparations

Make a photocopy of this handy checklist and place it on a bulletin board or on your refrigerator. Check off each item as you take care of it. As you check off the item, reread the section that discusses it so you don't accidentally leave anything out.

- ❏ Verify approval for extended sick leave from work with boss.
- ❏ Verify arrangements for blood donors, if any.
- ❏ Review which medicines and/or supplements to take before and after surgery with the surgeon.
- ❏ Discontinue medications and supplements per surgeon's instructions.
- ❏ Stock up on postsurgery medication and supplements; pack if necessary.
- ❏ Make arrangements for postsurgery meals, including grocery shopping for approved foods.
- ❏ Purchase a blender or food processor, if necessary.
- ❏ Purchase snack-sized food-storage containers, if necessary.
- ❏ Purchase a pill crusher.
- ❏ Purchase a good thermometer.
- ❏ Purchase a notebook for record-keeping.
- ❏ Arrange for a suitable place to sleep.
- ❏ Keep loose clothing handy.
- ❏ Confirm arrangements for child care.
- ❏ Confirm arrangements for pet care.
- ❏ Place mail and newspapers on hold.
- ❏ Plan for the payment of bills.
- ❏ Do housekeeping.
- ❏ Make sure everything's running smoothly, especially the car.
- ❏ Update will or prepare living will, if necessary.
- ❏ Confirm arrangements for company in the hospital and at home.
- ❏ Confirm hotel reservations, if any.
- ❏ Practice coughing, deep-breathing, and leg-pumping exercises.
- ❏ Work on a useful technique for getting out of bed.
- ❏ Learn to think positively.
- ❏ Pack bags for hospital stay.

part of your life? If so, you wouldn't be reading this book. You know that this kind of overeating is the enemy—it is the thing you want and need to control, and it's one of the main reasons you are having the surgery. Therefore, follow *all* of your nutritionist's recommendations. Enjoy your "last meal" but don't stretch the limits of your presurgery diet.

YOUR PRESURGICAL HISTORY AND PHYSICAL EXAM (H&P)

Hospital regulations require that you undergo a history and physical (H&P) before being operated on. Although the time and place for this H&P will vary, it usually takes place in your surgeon's office one or more days before the surgery. In some cases, however, it may be performed the morning of your surgery at the hospital.

Bring along one or more of your support people, especially those who will be helping you during your recovery. In addition to all of the preparations they've made to understand the surgery and the process you'll be going through, have them read any additional information you receive at this appointment, including the discharge instructions you are expected to follow after you leave the hospital.

At your H&P, you will once again review all of your medical history with the doctor and undergo another physical examination. Make sure that you bring an *updated* list of all medications and supplements—prescription *and* over the counter—you are currently taking along with dosage information. Make sure you're clear on which medications you should stop taking before surgery; write down any instructions you receive. Earlier in the process, you prepared a list of your medical problems and any prior surgeries. Bring this list with you to this appointment, too.

If your surgeon has not done so previously, he will review the results of all of your most current lab tests, x-rays, and other studies with you during your H&P. Then, he will once again go over with you the particulars concerning the type of surgery you are scheduled to have, including the risks, benefits, and possible surgical complications. As always throughout this process, you will be encouraged to ask questions. If you have any outstanding questions, be sure that you've prepared a list of them in advance so you don't forget anything of importance that you wanted to ask.

In some weight-loss-surgery centers, you may be required at this point to take a true-or-false or a fill-in-the-blanks exam to show that you understand the surgery and what it means. Don't worry about failing this test. If you've read this book and have done your research, you are well prepared.

Following the H&P, you will need to sign an "Informed Consent" form. As mentioned earlier, this is a legal document stating that you understand everything you need and want to know about the proposed surgery and wish to proceed with the operation. (Remember, however, that you do have the right to refuse surgery up until you lose consciousness on the operating-room table.) Be sure to read the "Informed Consent" form very carefully to be sure that you understand everything contained in it. If you don't, ask for clarification.

At any time leading up to your surgery, and especially during your H&P, if you have a cold, flu, or any sort of infection including of the abdominal wall, urinary tract, or chest, it is important that you report this to your surgeon as soon as you notice it. Also, if any symptoms appear just before surgery, it is crucial that you mention it to the hospital staff. For example, if you have a fever due to an infection that you don't mention, the surgeon may conclude that it is an indication of a surgical complication. This could lead to reoperation or a lot of unnecessary, expensive, and uncomfortable tests.

Whether or not your surgery will be rescheduled due to the infection depends upon how serious, or potentially serious, the infection is, in the examining physician's opinion. A very mild sore throat or a case of the "sniffles" probably won't be enough to warrant rescheduling the surgery. On the other hand, a full-blown infection of the urinary tract or lungs, for example, would most likely result in the surgery's postponement. Nevertheless, no matter how insignificant something seems to you, be sure to report it.

THE DAY BEFORE YOUR SURGERY

If you do not live a relatively short distance away from the hospital, you will need to stay at the hospital the night before your surgery in a special area of the hospital that, after 7 P.M. or so, is untended and you are "on your own" overnight. Alternatively, you may have to stay at a nearby hotel to avoid a long ride to the hospital the morning of your surgery.

Whether you're already at the hospital or not, there are certain things you will be instructed to do, or not do, for the twenty-four hours leading up to your surgery. The following sections should give you some idea of what to expect, but be sure that you understand and implement all of your surgeon's orders during these critical twenty-four hours.

Blood Work and Other Lab Tests

Since most states require certain tests to be done within forty-eight hours of surgery, you will probably undergo some more blood work the day before surgery, possibly at an independent lab. You may also be asked for a urine specimen. Do not eat or drink anything until your tests are complete. In fact, you may already be on liquids-only diet (see below). Don't rely on advice you receive from the staff at the lab regarding food or liquid intake since they won't necessarily be familiar with your surgeon's full testing schedule. When in any doubt about anything, call your surgeon's office for the correct information. Taking inaccurate advice may cause a delay in the surgery.

Consume Only Clear Liquids for 24 to 48 Hours Prior to Surgery

As mentioned earlier, you will be able to consume only clear liquids for twenty-four to forty-eight hours prior to surgery. Check with your surgeon's office to find out when you should switch to the liquids-only diet. You may find this information in your notes or in the surgeon's literature.

Use Your Incentive Spirometer and Perform Your Leg-Pumping Exercises

As mentioned earlier, deep-breathing exercises help prevent postsurgical lung problems. By this time, you will have received your incentive spirometer, a small plastic breathing apparatus. As a member of the hospital staff will show you, you use it by inhaling through a tube attached to a plastic cylinder. As you inhale, a movable disk or ball inside the cylinder will rise. The deeper you breathe, the higher the disk or ball will go. You'll want to get the ball or disk to go as high as you can. Each time you do the exercise, try to make the ball or disk rise higher than it did the last time. A plastic tab can be used to measure your progress. Take at least ten deep breaths with the incentive spirometer several times in the twenty-four hours preceding your surgery. (After surgery, you should use it, at least, every hour, or as instructed by your surgeon.)

It's also very important to practice your leg-pumping exercises quite frequently today (see page 119 for instructions).

Take a Laxative and Antibiotics If Instructed to Do So

Your surgeon will probably instruct you to take a laxative sometime during the day to prepare your digestive system for surgery and to reduce your chances of infection. You may also receive some special antibiotics to take for the same reason. Take notes of exactly what you have been instructed to do, and follow the directions very carefully.

Take a Cleansing Enema If Instructed to Do So

Sometime after you've taken the laxative, you will be instructed to take one or two cleansing enemas—an injection of liquid into the large intestine through the anus—to help empty your bowels and to help them work more easily after the surgery. If you will be traveling to the hospital or hotel, give yourself at least a couple of hours after taking the enema before getting into your car.

Wash With Antiseptic Soap in the Shower or Bath

You may be given a bottle of liquid antiseptic soap to shower or bathe with. If you did not receive special soap, just use regular antibacterial soap at least twice a day for two or more days before surgery. Make sure that you pay special attention to thoroughly cleansing your chest, including your breasts, abdomen, navel, and crotch areas. This helps prepare the skin for surgery and for the insertion of a catheter into your bladder with less risk of infection by reducing the number of bacteria normally found on your skin. Also, make sure that you do not use lotions or powder afterward.

Take Nothing By Mouth After Midnight Before Surgery

Do not take anything by mouth—not even liquids—after midnight before surgery. Be sure you are very clear about this, especially if you're sleeping at home the night before your surgery. If you're in the hospital, you can ask a nurse if you are unsure about what is allowed. This, of course, does not apply to the medications your surgeon has instructed you to take—just make sure it's absolutely clear to you what medications are, and are not, allowed, and have this information in writing to avoid problems.

THE DAY OF YOUR SURGERY

On the day of your surgery, you'll need to wake up very early—several hours in advance if you're not already at the hospital; otherwise, a couple of hours should do. After you check in to the hospital, a member of the nursing staff will process you. You'll need to fill out some paperwork and go over some of the hospital rules and services with the nurse. A health history may be taken from you once again, and you may receive even more instructions and information. This nurse or another hospital staff member will also make sure that all the necessary items are checked off on the hospital's checklist to prepare you for surgery. Any required last-minute tests will be performed this morning. In addition, there are a few other presurgical preparation you'll need to make the morning of your surgery, each of which is discussed below.

Cleansing Enema

Early this morning you may again receive, or be instructed to give yourself, a cleansing enema. This completes the preparation of your digestive system for surgery. Remember, if you are traveling to the hospital on the morning of your surgery, give yourself this enema at least one or two hours before leaving for the hospital.

Getting Down to Just You

Once you have some privacy, you will be given a hospital gown to change into. Remove all of your clothes, including your undergarments. Not wearing any of your own clothes to surgery helps reduce chances of infection. Also, remove any jewelry, glasses, wigs, hairpins, barrettes, contact lenses, makeup, dentures, nail polish (fingers and toes), and so on. All of these items could potentially interfere with your care while in surgery. In some cases, you may be permitted to wear your wedding ring or some other ring that's important to you into surgery. In this case, a member of the hospital staff can place surgical tape around it. (Leave any valuables with your family members for safekeeping, or better yet, leave them at home.)

Parting From Your Friends and Family

Depending upon the hospital's policy, one or two people may be permitted to stay with you for the few hours leading up to the surgery. At some point, however, you'll have to part ways. Remember to give your support person any valuables that may still be in your possession. This may be a very emotional time for all of you. Keep in mind that you've been preparing for this surgery for a very long time and you've had a chance to discuss all aspects of what's to come, so it shouldn't be necessary to have a long, drawn-out parting where you begin weighing the pros and cons of what you're about to do. Instead, focus on your feelings for each other, and know that your loved ones won't be far during the surgery. (See the inset "The Waiting Game" on page 128.)

Injection Before Surgery

Shortly before you are taken into the operating room, you may receive an injection that will help you relax but will not put you to sleep. Since this is the last time you'll have an opportunity to use the bathroom, it's important to empty your bladder immediately before this injection. (A member of the hospital staff will probably instruct you to do so.) Then, you will be taken to the operating-room holding area.

What Happens in the Operating-Room Holding Area

You will be brought on a bed or gurney to the operating-room holding area. Once there, your bed may temporarily be "parked" in a holding area until the operating room is ready for you. You will usually be in this holding area only for a short time.

The anesthesiologist will place a needle or small plastic tubing into one of your veins (in your arm, hand, neck, or under your collarbone) if it wasn't placed earlier. This tubing delivers fluids and medications you'll need before, during, and after surgery. Later, when you are able to drink enough fluid for your body's needs, this tubing will be removed.

Who's Who in the Operating Room

The people who work in the operating room (OR) wear special clothes, shoes, masks, and head coverings. You may see their eyes but little else of their faces. The surgeon and anesthesiologist will be accompanied by the surgeon's assistant, a scrub nurse (who prepares and passes instruments as requested and does other things necessary to help with the surgery itself), and one or two circulating nurses (who provide whatever help and support that the surgeon and anesthesiologist need before, during, and after your surgery).

The Waiting Game

During your surgery, your friends and family members should wait either in your assigned room or in the waiting room on your floor. If there's any question about where they should wait, suggest they check with a member of the hospital staff. During the surgery, one of the operating-room nurses will call to update them on the progress of the surgery. When the surgery is over, they will have a chance to speak with the surgeon. However, if they are not at the designated place when the surgeon calls or comes by, they'll miss what he has to say. If that happens, a nurse should be able to relay any essential information. Once your vital signs are stable and you have reasonably recovered from the anesthesia, your friends and family members will be permitted to see you.

What Goes On in the Operating Room

When the operating room is ready for you, you will be transferred from the bed or gurney onto the operating table, which is a padded, flat surface. You may have to wiggle yourself onto the table. You'll usually be provided with a foam cushion for your head to rest on. At this point, you may notice that the room is a bit chilly. The temperature is purposely kept a little lower than normal for comfort under the bright lights. The OR nurses may ask you to move your arms away from your sides and place them onto padded arm boards. Meanwhile, the anesthesiologist will usually fit an oxygen mask over your face to provide you with oxygen temporarily. When the anesthetic injected through your IV takes effect, you'll find that you become very relaxed and sleepy. At this point, the back of your throat may be sprayed with an anesthetic to allow a breathing tube, also called an *endotracheal tube,* to be passed into your windpipe in order to move oxygen and anesthesia gases in and out of your lungs while you are unconscious.

The passage of the tube through your mouth or nose usually takes less than half a minute, often just a few seconds. In some case, the anesthesiologist may have to perform what is called an *awake intubation,* especially in patients who have extremely large necks or who possibly have sleep apnea. This is done because of the increased difficulty of passing the tube into the patient's windpipe. The back of the throat is sprayed with anesthetic to make it numb and one of the nostrils is lubricated with a local anesthetic. Then, the tube is slowly and carefully passed into the windpipe. Most patients who undergo this procedure do not remember it.

Next, the surgeon will scrub your abdomen with a special soap and other solution in order to reduce the chances of your getting an infection in the surgical wound. Sterile drapes will then be placed over your abdomen. Then, the surgery begins. See Chapter 3 for an overview what takes place during the particular surgery you've chosen.

A few hours later, when the surgery is complete, all surgical equipment is removed from your abdominal cavity and the openings in the abdominal wall are closed. The skin may be sutured or stapled closed, sometimes with special tape, plastic, or gauze dressings depending on the surgeon's preferences. If drains or special tubes are placed, they are sewn to the skin and dressed or taped as well.

Anesthesia gases are then turned off and you will start to "come out of" the anesthesia. Sometimes this happens quickly enough to allow the anesthesiologist to remove your breathing tube right away. Sometimes, however, the anesthetic medicine and gases are slow to come out of your body's tissues, keeping you asleep a longer time. In this case, the breathing tube will probably be removed in the recovery room. If, however, you do not take deep enough breaths or if you have severe sleep apnea, the tube may remain in place for a while longer, sometimes overnight, with your breathing assisted by a machine called a *ventilator*. If this is the case, just relax and let the ventilator do the work of breathing for you until you are able to breathe deeply enough so that you do not need any more help. In some cases, if you do need to be on a ventilator overnight and tend to move around a lot, your hands (and sometimes your feet) may be restrained to avoid your accidental removal of the breathing tube or IV lines. If this is necessary, you will be given medication to help you relax. Remember, also, that the tube will prevent you from talking during this time. If you need to communicate something important, the nursing staff can help you write a note on piece of paper backed by a clipboard.

The Recovery Room, PACU, and ICU

When the surgery is over, you will most likely be taken to the recovery room—or to the post-anesthesia care unit (PACU). It will take about two to three hours for you to fully wake up from the anesthesia. You may feel a bit confused at first, but this is normal. About this time, your friends and family will be informed that your surgery is over. Your family members or friends will most likely not be permitted in the recovery room or the PACU, as this could interfere with other patients' privacy. In some cases, patients are placed in the intensive care unit (ICU) for the first twenty-four to forty-eight hours following surgery. This is almost always a precautionary measure and usually shouldn't be anything to be alarmed about. (For more information on what goes in the recovery room, the PACU, and the ICU, see the section "The Surgery Is Over—Now What?" in the next chapter.)

CONCLUSION

This chapter helped you prepare for your hospital stay and gave you some idea what to expect for the twenty-four to forty-eight hours leading up to your surgery. You've certainly come a long way since the beginning of this book, but your journey is only half over. There will be many difficult times ahead but also many benefits. Being familiar with what you can expect will make overcoming any difficulties you're about to face a little easier. The next chapter explains what to expect immediately after your surgery.

CHAPTER 8

*W*HAT TO EXPECT IMMEDIATELY AFTER SURGERY

Your long-awaited surgery is now over. When you wake up from the anesthesia, you'll probably be a little scared but full of anticipation. Or maybe you might wonder to yourself, "What have I done?" Don't be alarmed. Neither reaction is unusual. As the days pass, chances are you'll find yourself becoming excited about your future and you'll start thinking, "I'm on my way!"

From the tubes and wires, pain and the need for medication, and that new sensation of feeling "full" to preparing to check out of the hospital, this chapter covers much of what you will experience from the time you wake up from surgery until you are discharged. At the end of the chapter, you'll find a checklist to help you keep track of things to take care of before you leave the hospital. As you'll soon learn, these are important details, both major and minor.

THE SURGERY IS OVER—NOW WHAT?

After surgery, most patients are taken to the recovery room or the post-anesthesia care unit (PACU) for close observation until they fully regain consciousness. Many people wake up from the anesthesia while they are still on the operating-room table. Others wake up somewhat later in the recovery room or PACU. It's normal to feel confused and groggy and perhaps a little frightened as you start to become aware of your surroundings. If you've prearranged it, you will wake up to the sound of your positive-reinforcement audiotape. This may help you feel more at ease. (See the inset "Positive-Reinforcement Messages" on page 132.)

The tube that was inserted in the operating room will be removed from your windpipe when the nurse is satisfied that you are breathing and moving well enough to safely remove it. The removal is usually swift and painless with, at the most, a little gagging.

Once you appear to be in satisfactory condition, you will be either transferred to a regular room, to a "step down unit," or to the intensive care unit (ICU). Your surgeon will decide among these options based upon standard procedure, her professional judgment, and your particular case. If you are taken to the ICU after your surgery, you will be watched closely by a nurse who usually has only two or three patients to look after. If you are taken to a step down unit, the staff there will watch you almost as closely as the ICU nurse.

After surgery, you will have tubes and wires attached to your body for many different reasons. The purpose of the medical equipment and devices is discussed in some detail later in the chapter. Meanwhile, any pain you're feeling will need to be dealt with. The following section discusses pain management in the hospital.

Positive-Reinforcement Messages

Some surgeons provide their patients with motivational audiotapes for use after surgery, and even during surgery. Such tapes usually contain a series of important messages about coughing, deep breathing, moving, pain medicine, self-image, anti-smoking (if necessary), and other information that should hasten and improve your recovery. If your surgeon doesn't provide such a tape, you can make one yourself.

You can arrange to have your tape played for you when the surgery is over, or even during the surgery itself. After hitting play and checking the volume on the tape player, the nurse or other OR staff member will fit the headphones over your ears. (Remember, you need to have the audiotape and a continuous-loop or automatic-reverse tape player brought with you to the OR if you choose to use such a tape.)

At our center, we provide our patients with a set of "InThinity" audiotapes. With our set of tapes, a note on tape 1 instructs the OR staff member to insert it into the tape player. She will allow it to play for you during the surgery and will leave it on until you wake up. The positive-reinforcement messages on the tape are repeated over and over again so that you can "absorb" them while you are in the anesthetized state. Tape 2 is designed to be played at least once a day after surgery until your weight loss levels off, or for about

PAIN MANAGEMENT

As mentioned earlier, open weight-loss surgery requires a six- to twelve-inch incision in your abdomen while laparoscopic surgery requires multiple, usually one-inch or less, incisions. Therefore, the pain from open weight-loss surgery is generally more intense and lasts longer than that from laparoscopic surgery.

If you remain still, you may not feel any pain, but then, as you start moving around, you'll notice the discomfort—that is, if you haven't already been given pain-relieving medication. From time to time, your nurse will check on you and will usually ask how much pain you're experiencing on a scale of 0 (no pain) to 10 (unbearable pain). Be sure to let the nurse know the level of the worst pain you are feeling. For example, if you had severe back pain before surgery, this pain may be more intense than the pain you're feeling in your abdomen. Therefore, you would give the nurse the number that best describes your back pain.

---

a year. Thereafter, it should be played three or so times a week or any time additional reassurance is needed. It contains messages of self-assurance and positive feelings. Our patients who have used the tapes find that they helped them adjust to their new lives during and after massive weight loss.

A poster with a message relevant to the tape is provided along with the InThinity cassettes. Any tapes your surgeon provides may also come along with a poster. Posters with positive messages hung where you can see them often can help smooth your recovery. You can hang these posters on the walls in your hospital room and later at home for a constant reminder to maintain a positive outlook and to carry out important tasks.

You and your family might want to make posters at home before your surgery. Kids, especially, will enjoy this craft project. Some of the most important things for these posters to read include:

• Cough!	• Take deep breaths!	• Think thin!	• Smile!
• I am strong!	• I am complete!	• I am in control!	• I am great!

And, so you are! The sooner you take these statements into the center of your being the better. The more you see these messages, hear them, and repeat them to yourself, the sooner you will believe them. Be sure to take advantage of this aid to complete recovery.

You may feel some pain in some other places, too. The drains and tubes that are hooked up to your body may cause pain and irritation at the site of insertion. Also, if you've had open surgery, you may feel pain under your ribs, resulting from the use of a surgical instrument known as a *retractor*, which holds the abdomen open during surgery and also pulls your lower-most ribs up toward your shoulders. If you've had laparoscopic surgery, you may feel pain in your left shoulder, resulting from irritation to the undersurface of the diaphragm. No matter which type of surgery you've had, it is very important to report any shoulder pain to your nurse and/or surgeon since it may be due to a serious problem. Particularly, if you had open surgery, it may signal a leak from your stomach, which may prompt the taking of urgent x-rays to check for this possibility.

Narcotics are the main pain-relieving medications you will receive to help control your pain after surgery. Too much narcotic pain medication, however, can seriously slow, or even stop, your breathing. Very slow, shallow breathing can put you at risk for pneumonia. This is even more likely if you also have obstructive sleep apnea. Similar problems can occur in people with asthma or shortness of breath with very little effort or other lung conditions. Also, if you are super-morbidly obese, you are in greater danger of developing lung problems because your size makes it more difficult to take deep enough breaths after surgery.

Narcotics may also slow the movement of your intestines, delaying the passage of gas from your rectum or having a bowel movement. If frequent doses of narcotics are used for too long, this bloating and constipation can persist for days. As a result, your abdomen may swell, sometimes accompanied by cramping pain, nausea, vomiting, and belching.

For these reasons, your surgeon and nurses will give you only enough pain-relieving medication to control your pain and make it more bearable; therefore, some pain may still persist. Keep in mind that they are not deliberately making you suffer with the pain. They need to avoid giving you so high a dose of narcotics that it creates problems with your breathing, bowel activity, or worse. On the other hand, they'll want to make sure that they give you enough medication so that the pain does not stop you from coughing, breathing deeply, or moving around to help your recovery. Speak openly and honestly about the pain you're experiencing so they can make this determination.

Many people expect the pain medication to make *all* of their pain go away. Some even ask for additional pain medication to help them sleep. Due to the dangers of narcotics, including those mentioned above, you can surely understand why this is not the proper use for additional pain medication. Therefore, in order to avoid serious problems, only use the pain medication for *unbearable* pain. However, don't be so concerned about the side effects that you avoid using it completely in cases when you really do need it.

Some surgeons may give you non-narcotic anti-inflammatory medication for bone, joint, and/or muscle aches and pains. This medication, which does not slow your breathing, may work to relieve pain by itself. When given with the narcotic pain medication, it can enhance its effectiveness. However, some surgeons are cautious about giving this medication because it can interfere with blood clotting.

The pain from surgery should last for only a few days and will usually resolve sooner if you've had laparoscopic surgery. By the time they are discharged from the hospital, most people who have undergone weight-loss surgery require little, if any, pain medication. Nevertheless, a prescription for pain medication is usually written just in case.

Depending upon your individual needs, the method of pain-medication delivery may vary. Let's take a look at the various forms of delivery.

The Patient–Controlled Analgesia (PCA) Pump, or the "Pain Pump"

In some cases, your surgeon will order a PCA pump for you, commonly called the *pain pump*. This allows you to give yourself pain medication intravenously with the push of a button on a hand-held device every six or so minutes, depending upon the type of medication. If you push this button sooner than six or so minutes after your last dose, it is programmed to prevent you from receiving medicine, and nothing will happen. This "lock-out period" is meant to prevent you from getting an overdose of medicine by pushing the button too often. Also, you may be allowed only so many doses every two, three, or four hours and can be locked out for this reason as well. The first dose from the pump, called the *loading dose,* is usually somewhat higher than the doses that follow. Once you have some of the medicine in your body, the next dose, though lower, ought to be about as equally effective. The specific dosage details will vary depending upon your surgeon's orders. Your nurse can share the exact details with you if you ask.

The main advantage of the PCA pump is that you are able to get pain-relieving medication when you need it without having to call for the nurse. Make sure you pay attention to this *important warning:* Do *not* let anyone else push the PCA pump button for you. If you are too drowsy or have fallen asleep and are unable to push the button yourself, another dose administered by someone else could result in an overdose, perhaps enough to make you stop breathing.

If the pain pump does not help relieve your pain to the point where it is bearable, your nurse may be able to give you more medication. If permitted, she'll only give it to you if you appear relatively alert and your blood pressure and breathing rate are normal.

Pain Injections

If you don't have access to pain pump, a nurse will need to administer your pain medication. It may be injected into a tube leading to your vein or by a needle directly through your skin into your buttock, thigh, or upper-arm muscle. You may actually receive two injections—one for nausea and the other for pain. These medicines often work together to relieve your pain even more effectively than the pain medication alone. (By the way, some antinausea medicine may be given as a rectal suppository.)

Epidural Anesthesia

In some cases, you may receive epidural anesthesia. In this case, the anesthesiologist places a plastic tube through a needle inserted into your lower back. The pain medication is injected through this tube by a pump during surgery and for the first several days following surgery. When it works properly, most people appreciate its effectiveness at taking care of almost all of the postsurgical pain. However, there are some downsides to epidural anesthesia. First, the anesthesiologist may have problems properly inserting the needle and tube, which can be uncomfortable and can take extra time in the operating room. Second, the tube may accidentally fall out, may leak, or otherwise may not work correctly. Third, after surgery your nursing unit may run out of the replacement cartridges since this type of pain medication is not usually stocked on the floors. However, if epidural anethesia is routinely used at a certain hospital for their weight-loss surgery patients, chances are good that these problems will not occur.

Oral Pain Medication

As your discharge from the hospital nears and you are able to take liquids by mouth, your pain medication will likely be given orally every three to four hours. There are many different types of pain medications on the market, and different surgeons prefer to use different ones. Whatever the choice, we strongly recommend that this pain medication be in a liquid form or that it be crushed and mixed into a liquid. Taking your medication this way should prevent it from getting stuck in a fold or irregularity in your stomach pouch, where it could rest on the stomach lining and possibly cause an ulcer or irritation. If you have any concerns, speak with your surgeon.

WHAT THE TUBES AND WIRES ARE ALL ABOUT

When you start to regain consciousness after surgery, you'll discover various tubes and wires connected to different parts of your body. By learning about them in the following sections, you will know not to be alarmed, as they are all necessary and will aid in your recovery. It's important not to "test" or pull on them, since you may accidentally disconnect one. And now that you're partially or fully awake, reinsertion may be uncomfortable at the very least.

Oxygen–Delivery Device

Soon after you wake up, you'll discover that you are wearing an oxygen mask or that a plastic tube with prongs has been inserted into each of your nostrils. Whatever the case, this is providing your body—especially your stomach and intestines—with extra oxygen to help it heal. You'll continue to receive extra oxygen for as long as your surgeon feels you need it—sometimes up to two or more days following surgery. If you have sleep apnea, your surgeon may determine that you'll need to use the oxygen-delivery device while you're sleeping, perhaps both day and night; sometimes this

Don't Forget Your Breathing and Coughing Exercises

While you are awake, you will need to take deep breaths ten times every hour with your incentive spirometer to keep your lungs fully inflated to help prevent pneumonia. You will usually find that, as a result of breathing deeply, you will have to cough; if not, try to make yourself cough at least once or twice to clear whatever secretions you may have in your upper airways or way back in your throat. Hold a cushion or folded blanket (your "cough pillow") over your wound while taking deep breaths or coughing to lessen the discomfort.

may replace your breathing machine for several weeks at home. Other patients who have low oxygen levels that persist after surgery may even need to go home with the oxygen-delivery device, as well; this seems to be more common in areas of the country that are thousands of feet above sea level.

Nasogastric (NG) Tube

When you wake up from surgery, you might notice a small plastic tube coming out of your nose. This is most likely a nasogastric (NG) tube. The NG tube is a flexible plastic tube that is inserted through your nose and into your stomach pouch during surgery. A suction device at the other end of the tube removes the contents of your new stomach pouch to keep it empty for a day or so after surgery as well as to prevent nausea and vomiting and to reduce the chance of a leak. While the NG tube is in, the nurse will flush it occasionally to make sure the passage is clear and then reconnect it to the suction device. Don't be alarmed if fluid is not draining constantly from the tube; it will work as needed. The NG tube will be removed as early as possible, usually the day after surgery; however, some surgeons remove the NG tube soon after surgery, so don't be surprised if you do not have one when you awaken. While the tube is in place, you are usually not allowed to eat or drink. This is partly to prevent your small stomach pouch from becoming overloaded soon after surgery.

Abdominal Drain

When you wake up from surgery, you may notice an abdominal drain leading from your abdomen. This plastic tube was placed there to drain out any fluids that could collect within your abdominal cavity, including fluid from your stomach if, in the rare event, a leak develops. Not all surgeons use a drain after surgery, so don't be surprised if you do not have one. This tube is usually left in place for several days or until the drainage from your abdomen is less than 1 ounce per twenty-four hours.

Subcutaneous Drain

In some cases, your surgeon may place a subcutaneous drain under your skin to prevent the collection of fluid, called a *seroma*. If this is done, you'll notice one or two tubes coming out of your incision or elsewhere on your skin. Unlike the abdominal drain, the purpose of these drains is to remove fluid from under your skin, *outside* the abdomen. In about one-third of the cases, serum (sometimes blood-stained) will drain out through this tube(s), perhaps for days. Don't panic if you fall into this category. The drainage will eventually stop. Only occasionally will a wound need to be opened wider for better drainage or for treating a possible infection.

Gastrostomy Tube (G–Tube)

As explained in Chapter 3, some weight-loss surgeons place a tube—known as a *gastrostomy tube,* or G-tube—into the bypassed stomach. It is much more commonly placed in open surgery than in laparoscopic surgery. The reason for the placement of the G-tube is that the pylorus—the muscle at the bottom of the stomach—sometimes spasms and prevents the stomach juices from draining out through the bottom end of the stomach. When the upper end of the stomach has been stapled shut, the G-tube functions as another way for the juices to leave the stomach to prevent it from inflating.

This tube is not removed before you leave the hospital; instead, it is usually removed several weeks after surgery during an office visit with the surgeon. By this time, there should be no risk of muscle spasm. If necessary, your surgeon may leave the G-tube in longer for the purpose of providing medication or nourishment through it. If this is the case, the nurses at the hospital will usually show you to handle the tube at home. This may involve opening the tube and letting it drain out two or more times daily.

In some cases, you'll need to flush the tube with a large syringe, which should be given to you before you leave the hospital. You'll be asked to record the amount of fluid that drains out. If more than a cup (8 ounces or 240 cc) drains out of the G-tube, you must inform your surgeon's office promptly and ask for further instructions.

Heart Monitor

After surgery—especially if you're in the ICU—your heart rate will probably be monitored with an EKG machine. If you are being monitored by an EKG machine, small adhesive electrodes, which are completely painless, will be attached to your chest, wrists, or ankles. Wires then connect the electrodes to a monitor in your room. If your heart rate should become abnormal, the monitor will sound an alarm to alert the nurses of a potential problem.

Oxygen–Sensor Clip

A small plastic clip may be placed over one of your fingers or on your ear-lobe. Attached to this clip is a wire leading to a machine that keeps track of your heart rate and the level of oxygen in your blood. If the screen on the machine indicates low levels of oxygen, you will need additional oxygen or further attention by a respiratory technician, nurse, or doctor. It is especially important that this machine remain on at all times, even when you are sleeping or just napping.

These machines sometimes malfunction, causing an incessant beeping. Contact the nurses' station immediately to report a machine that beeps incessantly. Do *not* turn off the machine to stop the beeping. The beeping may actually be indicating that you require more oxygen.

Intravenous (IV) Fluid Tubing

As mentioned earlier, before surgery, a needle attached to a tube may have been placed into one of your veins, usually in your arm or hand. The needle is then taped in place, and you will almost forget it is present after a while. Fluid, antibiotics, and anesthetic are delivered through the IV. After surgery, the IV will remain to ensure that your body receives enough fluids. It will usually remain in place until your bowels begin to function and you are able to eat and drink enough to nourish your body. Take special care not to accidentally disconnect the IV tube.

Alternatively, your IV may have been placed into one of the large veins in your neck or under your collarbone, probably while you were under anesthesia. This type of IV is generally more secure and allows fluids to flow into your body very quickly if you need them. This also leaves your hands and arms free.

Arterial Line to Watch Your Blood Pressure

In some cases, a small plastic tube will be placed into one of your arteries, usually the radial artery, which is located in the wrist. This tube is attached to a monitoring device that is used to monitor your blood pressure during surgery and in the recovery room or ICU. Also, blood can be drawn through this tube. Before you are transferred to a regular room, this line will be removed.

Foley Catheter (Tube in the Bladder)

During surgery, a small tube called a *Foley catheter* is usually inserted into your bladder to keep it empty of urine and to make sure your kidneys are working properly. It is usually removed the day after surgery. However, if you are putting out too little urine, it may be left in for a few extra days.

Most surgeons prefer to get the catheter out early to encourage you to get out of bed, to make it less likely you will get a urinary tract infection, and to hasten your recovery.

If you develop burning or stinging when you pass urine, be sure to tell your nurse since this may indicate an infection.

After the catheter is removed, you will be expected to get out of bed to use the toilet or a bedside commode. Unless you are pretty free of pain and walking well, you should insist on having an extra-wide bedside commode available for your use.

Inflatable Boots

To help prevent your blood from clotting, you may find yourself wearing inflatable boots on your legs and sometimes on your thighs. In fact, you may have been wearing these boots during your surgery.

The boots inflate for about twelve seconds every minute. They massage your calves, causing your blood flow to be less sluggish, and thereby reduce the formation of blood clots. The air pressure in these boots is a little less than half of that used to inflate a blood-pressure cuff, and should not be uncomfortable.

Wound Dressings

Wound dressings for incisions made during open surgery will be larger than those for laparoscopic surgery. You may have wide elastic tape over the surgical wound or just small, adhesive bandages and/or plastic coverings, or something else. A surgeon's choice of dressing generally comes from her experience with caring for surgical incisions. Follow all of your surgeon's rules with regard to your wound dressing. Also, if you notice drainage from the wound, bring it to your nurse's attention.

WHAT ELSE TO EXPECT
DURING YOUR STAY AT THE HOSPITAL

Okay, so you're fully awake, you've been transferred to your regular room, and you're ready for the remainder of your hospital stay. Family, friends, and members of the hospital staff will be coming and going from your room, and you may, at times, feel like you have no privacy. At other times, you may crave company or just someone to talk to. You may experience some new sensations and undergo additional tests. This is all a normal part of your hospital stay. Being familiar with what else to expect while you're in the hospital can help you cope with the days ahead. Let's take a look at some of them.

Additional Blood Work

During your stay at the hospital, blood will be drawn from you, perhaps a few times. This blood work allows your surgeon and other hospital staff members to determine levels of things such as your hemoglobin—the oxygen-carrying part of the red blood cell—which may be low if you are becoming anemic; white blood cells, which, if elevated, may mean you have an infection or inflammation developing; sugar, which is sometimes elevated following surgical stress—not just in diabetics; and kidney and liver chemistry. If there is a problem with any of the results of your blood work, your surgeon will discuss these problems with you and/or your family members who may be present if you desire.

Visits from Specialists

If your medical condition is straightforward and you did not have any significant comorbidities, you may see only one or two specialists, including the nutritionist. If your case is more complex, however, you may be seen by several specialists who will help with your care during your stay in the hospital. Depending on their recommendations, you may undergo additional tests.

Getting Out of Bed and Moving Around

Your nurses and surgeon will give you some tips for moving around in bed, exercising your legs, and getting in and out of bed, which will be difficult and may be painful at first. These are important exercises that help your recovery. We usually recommend that patients get out of bed on the day of their operation with assistance. It's a good idea to walk in place (for about twenty steps) next to your bed, with one of your thighs touching the edge of the bed. This way, if you become unsteady, you can easily sit back down. After that first day, we usually recommend that the patient get up at least once per hour during waking hours. Also, since we can't stress it enough, it's important to breathe deeply, cough up any secretions, and use your incentive spirometer every hour during waking hours.

Also, an abdominal binder—a wide elastic compression garment that wraps around your abdomen—is usually provided by the hospital for your comfort when walking. (Or you may have been instructed to purchase an abdominal binder from a surgical supply store before your surgery.) This garment helps support the abdomen and relieves some of the pain when getting up after surgery. It should not be worn when you are sitting or lying down as it can restrict the amount of air that reaches your lungs. Some surgeons do not want their patients to use a binder, so do not use one unless you have your surgeon's permission.

Visits From Family and Friends

Although rules vary from hospital to hospital, you will usually be permitted two visitors, usually relatives, to visit with you at certain times of the day. Some hospitals may permit family members or friends to say with you during non-visiting hours, and some may even allow a spouse or other important person to stay overnight on a cot in your room. Since you know what hospital you'll be staying in, you can check on the hospital's visitors' policy beforehand.

If permitted, it's certainly nice to have help from a support person during your stay in the hospital. This person can help you get to the toilet, get ice chips for you, or provide you with anything else you might need. It's also comforting just to have someone with you. Having said that, anyone who will be staying with you and intends to help must be properly instructed by a nurse about what is permitted and what is not. If you are unsure about anything, don't hesitate to ask. Although well intentioned, a person who is not properly instructed on the do's and don'ts may inadvertently cause a problem.

Oxygen–Level Monitor

The oxygen-sensor clip was discussed on page 139. However, it bears repeating here, since oxygen levels in the blood can drop dangerously low after surgery, especially in morbidly obese patients. In most instances, the hospital staff cannot tell whether or not your oxygen level is normal by

No Smoking!

Smoking in the hospital is strictly forbidden. Aside from the dangers of first- and secondhand smoke and your need to breathe clean air, especially after surgery, smoking around pure oxygen is a serious fire hazard. If you or any of your visitors are smokers, you must comply with this rule for the safety and comfort of all concerned.

just looking at you. So be sure not to remove the oxygen-sensor clip on your finger or ear, if you've been fitted with one. And, as mentioned earlier, do not turn off the machine. In some cases, in addition to the monitor, blood gas samples may be taken from an artery in your wrist to determine your oxygen levels.

If you have been receiving additional oxygen due to low levels, your surgeon or other specialist will stop the oxygen once the concentration in your blood is high enough—one or more days after surgery.

If you have sleep apnea, you may have been using a CPAP or BiPAP machine prior to surgery. At this point, your surgeon may instruct you to start using it again. Be sure not to use it until you get permission. If you are in doubt, ask your surgeon.

Intestinal Gas

Adults normally swallow about fifty times an hour. Each time we swallow, we also swallow air. This is where most of the gas in our intestines comes from. Most of the air we swallow eventually passes out of the rectum as flatus, although sometimes it may come out as a "burp." However, it can cause gas pains, especially when more air is being swallowed than normal. This may happen during the first few days of your hospital stay, since you may swallow even more often due to nerves, and find that this is causing you intestinal distress.

One way to prevent gas pains due to excessive swallowing is to place a clean, capped pen or pencil lengthwise between your teeth and hold it there. This keeps your mouth open slightly, making it more difficult to swallow. This will reduce the amount of air you swallow. We recommend using this technique for a couple of days following surgery—except of course, when you're eating or drinking—to prevent your stomach from blowing

---

Passing Gas—A Good Sign of Your Recovery

When you begin to pass gas through your rectum instead of belching, that's a good sign of your recovery. When your bowels begin to go back to work, you may experience a few mild to moderate gas pains. This process will be aided by rectal suppositories and enemas, which will usually start to be administered about a day or two after surgery. Walking frequently also helps speed the process.

up with air and causing abdominal pain. While this sounds and may look unusual, this method really does work. We advise you to use this technique even before you really need it. Remember, a pen in the mouth is better than a pain in the abdomen.

Resuming Your Medication

Even before you start to eat or drink, you may start to take some medication by mouth, including those you were taking before your surgery, such as for high blood pressure or diabetes. Your surgeon will let you know, or will leave orders with the nurses, for when these medications should be resumed. As mentioned previously, we recommend that you do not take your medicines in pill form. Rather, they should be crushed or liquefied for the next six weeks. Speak to your nurse about crushing your tablets, and when you get home, use your pill crusher. Whole pills and capsules can get "hung up" in your new, narrow, stomach pouch and irritate the lining or even cause a deep ulcer. If you have any questions about the absorption of any of your medications in crushed form, be sure to discuss this with your surgeon or nurse.

Nausea and Vomiting

Even if you obey all the do's and don'ts, you may still experience frequent nausea or vomiting. This is no need for alarm since it occurs for a short time in about one-fourth to one-third of all patients following weight-loss surgery. However, be sure to inform the nurse and surgeon if you do feel nauseated. Once alerted, your surgeon may want to have x-rays taken to see if there is a problem. There are dozens of other reasons besides serious problems for nausea and vomiting. In almost all cases, the nausea and vomiting can be treated or allowed to resolve on their own in about one to three days. Only rarely will it take longer and need further treatment.

Depression

About 15 to 20 percent of our postsurgical patients develop depression while in the hospital or shortly after discharge. At least in some cases, it may be due to hormonal changes or the effects of some medications, including the anesthesia. The more obvious signs of depression include tiredness and/or sleeping all the time, not sleeping at night, an unwillingness to get out of bed, refusing to walk, hiding under the bed sheets, crying, irritableness, dissatisfaction, or an unhappy or sad demeanor. Many patients do not realize that they are depressed or may deny it. You may be one of them. It's important to consider the possibility and to be honest with yourself and the hospital staff. If you are feeling depressed, be sure to mention this to your nurse or surgeon. If a hospital staff member suspects that you are depressed, she will bring it to your surgeon's attention. Your surgeon may decide to prescribe antidepressants for you. If you had been taking anti-depressants prior to your surgery, you'll want to discuss restarting them as soon as possible with your surgeon.

PREVENTING BLOOD CLOTS AFTER SURGERY

After your surgery and continuing for about six weeks, the blood in your veins may be more likely to clot—especially in your legs, thighs, or pelvis. These clots can later travel to your lungs and cause a life-threatening situation. You and your surgeon can help to make this less likely to happen by taking a number of steps, which are discussed below.

Blood-Thinning Medication

You may receive small doses of blood-thinning medication such as heparin once or twice a day while in the hospital and, occasionally afterward, to help prevent blood clots. Like most treatments, your surgeon has to balance the risk of potential blood clots without blood-thinning treatment against the low risk of bleeding after surgery due to blood thinners.

Inflatable Boots

As mentioned earlier, inflatable boots are usually used to help prevent your blood from clotting. They work about 95 percent as well as blood-thinning medication. However, unlike this medication, the boots do not increase the risk of postsurgical bleeding. When you are able to get out of bed and walk around at least a dozen or more times per day, the boots will be removed. Therefore, it's up to you to "earn" their removal by increasing your activity each day.

Leg-Pumping Exercises

When the inflatable boots are removed, you'll need to get your leg-pumping exercises into high gear to prevent your blood from thickening. Following their removal and for the next six weeks, you'll need to pump your legs regularly. Do this exercise as often as you think about it—1,000 or so times each day.

Proper Positioning of Your Legs

Keep your legs up on a cushion or chair while sitting. You'll need to do this for the following six weeks. Like walking and your leg-pumping exercises, this will help the circulation in your legs and reduce the chances of complications such as leg swelling and blood clots. Also, do *not* cross your ankles or legs after surgery or for the following four to six weeks, since this can slow the blood flow in your legs.

Walking

Walking is one of the best ways to improve the blood circulation in your legs and throughout your body. While you are walking, your leg muscles squeeze the blood vessels that run through them. This helps send the blood back to your heart more efficiently.

CONTROLLING BLEEDING AFTER SURGERY

Any major abdominal surgery involves the risk of internal bleeding. If your hemoglobin—the oxygen-carrying part of the red blood cell—level falls by a fair amount and you become weak or there are major changes in your vital signs, your surgeon may decide to give you a blood transfusion or, more rarely, return you to the operating room to control the bleeding.

Before any additional surgery is performed, it is likely that x-ray, radioisotope, or scope studies will be taken to determine where the bleeding is coming from. More than likely, the source of bleeding will be from the area of the surgical staples or stitches, from a torn blood vessel in the abdominal wall (more common with laparoscopy), from a bleeding ulcer, or from the spleen, a blood-forming organ located above and to the left of the stomach. Sometimes ulcers with bleeding blood vessels can be injected with a substance that controls the bleeding, and surgery is therefore not necessary.

CHECKING YOUR PROGRESS WITH X-RAYS

In most cases, you'll recover a little bit each day while you're in the hospital. Of course, there's always a chance of a complication—for example, see the inset "A Swollen Abdomen—A Possible Sign of Complications" on page 148—but if you're like most people, you'll be on the road to recovery. Still, your surgeon will want to check on your progress. A day or two before you are discharged, you may be taken to the x-ray department for a CT scan or an upper GI series to make sure that everything is proceeding satisfactori-

A Swollen Abdomen— A Possible Sign of Complications

After surgery, your intestines may decide to lie down on the job and not move juices and liquids through your system as they normally would. As a result, your abdomen may become somewhat swollen, perhaps more tender or painful, and normal bowel sounds will be absent. You may also experience some nausea and/or vomiting. This condition is called *ileus.*

Ileus usually resolves quickly after oral medicines and liquids are withdrawn, a rectal suppository to encourage bowel movement is administered, and IV fluids and medicines are increased. In some cases, an x-ray may indicate that you have small bowel obstruction, also called *locked bowels,* in which the bowel is kinked or otherwise twisted, preventing food, liquid, or digestive juices from passing downward to the colon. Such a condition may require an emergency reoperation in about 2 percent of cases, even years after weight-loss surgery. If it is thought to be a small bowel obstruction, surgery is best done as soon as possible to avoid possible damage, or even death, of the obstructed bowel.

In the majority of cases, patients recover nicely. However, if this complication develops and you do require emergency surgery, your discharge from the hospital will be delayed and you will still be at risk of postsurgical complications.

ly. You may also have chest x-rays taken. (Chest x-rays are usually taken a few times after surgery, usually with a portable x-ray machine at your bedside.) Unfortunately, some super-morbidly obese patients are too large for the CT scanner or certain other x-ray machines, in which case, decisions about possible complications may have to be made without their use.

READY TO EAT AND DRINK?

Following surgery, you will receive nourishment intravenously for one to three or more days, depending upon the type of surgery you've had. When your surgeon feels you are ready to drink, she may order ice chips and/or water for you. If this goes down okay, you will probably be placed on a clear-liquid diet. This usually includes a small amount of flavored gelatin such as Jell-O, juice, and broth.

Do not try to drink everything on your tray all at once; in fact, you don't have to finish it all (see the inset "No More, Thanks!" below). Sip your liquids slowly, put your cup down, and wait about three minutes before your next sip. This is an important part of developing your new eating behavior. In the beginning, take thirty minutes to finish one ounce. Later, finish it in twenty minutes, then in ten minutes. Drinking liquids any faster than that is too fast.

We know of a few people who, despite their surgeon's orders, drank large amounts of water shortly after surgery. In some of these cases, the small stomach pouch burst open before proper healing had taken place as a result of this excessive intake. This allowed anything in the stomach pouch to flow into the clean abdominal cavity. This can cause a serious, life-threatening infection. In such a case, emergency surgery will usually be required to repair the damage, thereby complicating and prolonging time to recovery.

If you receive the wrong tray—one that contains solid foods or fluids you are not permitted to drink—do *not* consume any of the items on that tray, no matter how tempting. Inform the nurse immediately that you've been given the wrong tray. Also, beware of carbonated beverages. You will not be permitted to drink any carbonated beverages for the next six weeks

No More, Thanks!

You will probably find that there's more on your tray than you are able to drink. You don't have to finish it all. Take enjoyment in the new experience of pushing away leftovers. Smile and congratulate yourself for "joining" all those people who push their plates away when they feel full. Along with this, mentally picture all those good things you are going to be able to do as you get smaller and smaller—once again, give yourself a big, warm smile. You are on your way to really starting to like and love yourself and your new body. This is an enjoyable and important part of your new self.

Later, when you switch to solid food, you may be surprised that you can eat only one or two ounces of food before becoming full. Don't worry about wasting the leftovers. You are allowed—in fact, you're encouraged—to quit your membership in the "Clean Plate Club." Throwing away or storing excess food rather than eating it is one of the important habits you will need to develop. And, again, smile to yourself whenever you store or discard extra food because you're too full to eat it! Remind yourself how sweet it is.

or more; the carbon dioxide gas that gives the drink its fizz may danger-ously raise the pressure in your small stomach pouch and cause damage. In fact, some surgeons advise their patients to avoid carbonated beverages for up to a year.

When you show that you can tolerate clear liquids without problems, you may be advanced to a full liquid diet. In addition to the clear liquids, this will include milk and milk products, other liquids, cream soups, and very thin hot cereals. However, your surgeon may skip dairy products, or just add small amounts, especially if you have experienced lactose intoler-ance—an inability or reduced ability to process milk sugar. Most people, even those with lactose intolerance, can consume small amounts of dairy products without any problem.

Once you are able to tolerate the full liquids diet, you may be advanced to a diet that includes puréed foods. Keep in mind that surgeons handle their patients' food and liquid intake after surgery in many different ways. The type of surgery you've had also factors in to how soon puréed foods are started. Some surgeons will advance your diet quickly while you're still in the hospital; others will keep you on liquids for another ten to fourteen days. Again, this depends a great deal on the type of surgery you've had. The most important thing here is that you do *exactly* what your surgeon has instructed you to do. If you are unsure, speak to your surgeon or nutrition-ist and take notes.

When you do begin the puréed diet, wait about thirty minutes after drinking before eating the puréed food. Then, wait another half hour before drinking liquids. Without this waiting period, the liquids and purées have a tendency to "stack up" on each other in the stomach pouch, causing feed-back. Don't try it—you won't like it. Also, when eating puréed foods, remember to eat only from one-ounce cups (see the inset "Your New Din-nerware" on page 151). And as with your liquids, don't eat the one ounce any faster than in ten minutes. Chew the purée thoroughly, especially in the front of your mouth, at least twenty times. Wait three minutes between mouthfuls.

Don't forego your liquids when you've started eating puréed foods. If you do not drink enough liquid, you could become dehydrated or consti-pated and even develop kidney problems. Therefore, by the time you're discharged, you need to be drinking a minimum of 40 ounces each day. That's *forty* one-ounce cups.

Not everyone's diet advances from liquids to solid food at the same rate. By six weeks to three months after surgery, you should be able to eat

---

Your New "Dinnerware"

Using one-ounce medicine cups as well as thin straws and sampler-sized spoons for your food and liquids will help you change your eating behavior. These items are small like your new stomach pouch and can protect you from making the mistake of swallowing too much food or liquid at one time, which can damage your stomach pouch. They also make it easier to keep track of the number of ounces you take in each day. It is important that you continue to use them even at home for your purées until you are on a solid diet. If you do not receive these smaller-sized items with your meals, ask your nurse to provide them. Later, you might find that children's "sippy" cups come in quite handy for taking small sips throughout the day.

---

a wide variety of solid foods, in small portions of course. However, some people may have problems with certain foods a year after surgery or even permanently. If something does not agree with you, make a note of it and avoid it for a few weeks. Later, you may want to try the food again in an even smaller amount. As an individual, you will have your own tolerances and intolerances, likes and dislikes. Most people, for instance, have some foods that they just can't stand and other foods they want. Sometimes, you may prefer a type of food after surgery that you didn't like before. Therefore, when you are finally permitted to eat solid food, you will have to experiment to determine what's right for you. Since many of our patients find that they have dramatic changes in their food preferences, you might be surprised by what you like and dislike.

Postsurgical Nutrition

At some point before you are discharged, you will probably see your nutritionist. She will go over with you all the dietary recommendations and related matters. If you don't know if such a visit has been scheduled, ask your nurse. If such a visit has not been scheduled, speak to your surgeon about arranging one.

As part of this meeting, the nutritionist will stress the importance of protein intake. The weight loss following surgery should come from a reduction in fat not muscle. To prevent the loss of muscle and to preserve your strength, you'll want to take in at least 60 grams of protein a day within a few days following surgery (we recommend 80 grams to be on the safe side). The nutritionist will provide you with more exact recommendations as well as dietary suggestions and advice on protein supplement products. Remember to eat your protein foods before you eat anything else so that you don't fill up on other, less important, foods. (Chapter 9 covers some important dietary recommendations in detail.)

Keeping Score of What Goes In and What Goes Out

Keep a written record of the amount of liquid, including water, and food you consume each day. It's like keeping score at a ball game—draw a small line for each ounce you drink; then, when you drink your fifth ounce, place a diagonal line through the four lines. Do the same for food. A good goal is at least 40 ounces of food and/or liquids every twenty-four hours. You'll want to "keep score" of your protein intake each day as well.

You'll also need to keep track of your bowel movements if they become too frequent. This is not unusual especially with people who have had their gallbladders removed or whose food and common limbs are shorter than they would be with regular gastric bypass procedures. However, discuss any frequent, or very watery, stools with your surgeon, who will help you control them better with medicine or other treatment, if necessary.

In some types of surgery—generally malabsorptive procedures—you will have some liquid stools, which will be darkly hued due to bile drainage from your liver. After you start eating, your bowel movements will become more regular (usually once or twice a day) but will be somewhat mushy and yellow-colored. Also, you may have some foul-smelling gas and bowel movements due to partially digested fats in your large intestine. While this does not bother some people much, you may want to use a deodorant spray, such as Ozium, and also reduce the amounts of fat in your diet.

GETTING READY TO GO HOME

If you've had open weight-loss surgery, you will have been in the hospital for about four to six days, assuming there were no complications. For laparoscopic surgery, one to three days is the norm. As long as everything is satisfactory—that is, you're able to eat and drink, you're walking around, and all your tests are in the normal range—you will be discharged on schedule. If you are from out of town and will be staying at a local hotel, you'll be visiting your surgeon's office every few days, and she will clear you for travel when it's determined that you're well enough to make the ride home.

Double check with your surgeon about any medication you should or should not be taking. Be sure to write everything down. At this point, you should already have a good idea of what is expected, since you so diligently did your homework as recommended in earlier parts of this book.

There's a lot to remember as you prepare yourself for your journey home, so we've prepared the checklist below to help you make sure all your bases are covered.

Checklist for Going Home

❏ Receive understandable instructions on how to care for and manage any remaining tube(s) and wound dressing.

❏ Confirm transportation arrangements from the hospital.

❏ Confirm hotel reservations, if any.

❏ Go over the list of all permitted medications and their dosages.

❏ Get prescriptions for pain and antinausea medication, antibiotics, and any other medications the surgeon has prescribed for use at home.

❏ Verify that prescriptions have been filled or make arrangements to have them filled.

❏ Make a list of all follow-up appointments with the surgeon; schedule the necessary appointments if they haven't been made.

❏ Put the surgeon's office and emergency numbers in a safe, accessible place.

❏ Find out when to call the surgeon for an emergency and when to go to the emergency room. Ask the surgeon for an emergency-notice card, or Med-Alert card (see page 166).

❏ Gather all personal items, including any inspirational posters and tape player, and any necessary medical supplies.

❏ Gather together all written instructions and keep in a safe place.

❏ Ask for a supply of one-ounce cups, sampler-sized spoons, and cocktail straws. Ask the surgeon for a special meal card (see page 174).

❏ Remember to say "congratulations" for taking these first steps on the journey toward weight loss, increased quality of life, and, most important, better health.

THE RIDE HOME

If you live close to the hospital, the ride home shouldn't be too bad. If you must ride for several hours in a car, bus, or plane to get home, you may find all the bumps and vibrations somewhat painful, even after having spent a few days at a nearby hotel. You can ask your surgeon for pain medication in order to avoid some of this travel-associated discomfort. Most surgeons will be willing to order a shot of pain medication just before you embark on your journey home. However, you must remember to ask for it if you think you need it.

If you're riding in a car, take frequent stops along the way, if possible, every half hour or so. Get out of the car and walk around for at least three minutes or more. If you are on a bus or airplane, get up from your seat and walk the aisles for a few minutes every so often when permitted. Also, do some leg-pumping exercise if room permits. While you are walking, be sure to take at least ten deep breaths. Remember, deep breathing will help prevent lung problems. Also, it's a good idea to avoid eating anything before the ride, since your stomach is still healing and won't be completely settled. Sip some water to stay hydrated.

CONCLUSION

This chapter has taken you from what to expect immediately after surgery up until the time you are discharged. The things that will likely occur during your hospital stay will no longer be such a mystery to you. While it's virtually impossible to cover every experience you will have, this chapter covered quite a bit of it. Likewise, the chapters ahead will give you a good idea of what to expect in the coming weeks and months.

CHAPTER 9

ℐOUR ARRIVAL HOME AND THE FIRST SIX MONTHS

A ll the planning is over. The surgery is over. And you're back home. Although you are getting much closer to your long-term goals, there's still much to keep you busy in terms of recovery and building your exciting new life. To help, this chapter will give you a good idea of what you can expect for the next six months and what you can do to ensure a speedy and full recovery. It provides some important details about your new diet and other lifestyle changes, as well as important advice about how to care for yourself. This should be first and foremost on your mind. So, let us begin this chapter with some important recommendations and suggestions for a healthier future.

FOCUS ON YOUR HEALTH

Recovering and benefiting from weight-loss surgery takes a lot of hard work. You'll have to make your health your first priority for life, not only to take care of the new you, but also to avoid medical complications that can occur even long after your surgery. Now that you're on your own, you'll discover just how physically committed you must be to your altered anatomy. You'll need to focus your mind on your new drinking and eating program to make your surgery and the ongoing changes in your body work best for you. This is a very serious commitment. For now, you must put everything else in your life second to your body's hourly and daily needs in order to realize your long-term weight-loss goals and to minimize surgical risk, costs, and pain. If you do not put your well-being first and wind up suffering from complications as a result, those who depend on you—your children, spouse, friends, coworkers, and others—will also suffer. In short, whether you like it or not, stick to the rules! To help you take care of yourself during your recovery, take heed of the advice in the following sections. These sections are followed by specifics about your new eating plan and exercise regimen.

Taking It Easy

When you first get home, it will probably feel like you've been gone a long time. So much has happened since you left for the hospital, but it really was just a relatively short time ago. Your house should be in good order because of all the preparations you made before you left for the hospital, and hopefully you'll have a support person on hand to help with the chores. That's good, because you'll likely be very tired as a result of everything you've been through. Although you'll probably feel like you should get right back into the swing of things, it's important not to be too active for the next forty-eight hours or so. Thereafter, continue to take it easy before gradually resuming your normal routine. While it's important to walk around a dozen or so times each day, don't overdo it. Listen to your body; if it says stop, then stop. This is an essential time to rest and take care of your body.

Climbing Stairs

If you have to climb stairs soon after surgery, we recommend that you go up and down only a maximum of three times a day for the first ten to fourteen days. When you do need to take the stairs, take "baby steps"—that is, place both feet on one step before going on to the next one. To prevent accidents, avoid climbing stairs as much as possible until your strength has returned.

Sleeping Arrangements

If you've done your homework, you've already set up temporary sleeping quarters for yourself on the ground floor. As mentioned previously, you may be most comfortable sleeping on a recliner for a week or two. In some cases, your surgeon will have ordered a hospital bed for your use at home. Remember, waterbeds are not suitable for use after surgery as it is too much of a struggle to get in and out of them.

Lifting

Do not lift, push, or pull anything with a force or weight greater than ten to fifteen pounds for the first *six weeks* after your surgery. Thereafter, do not lift, push, or pull anything heavier than twenty-five pounds for six months. After six months, you will not have any weight restrictions unless you have a problem such as a hernia. Check with your surgeon just to make sure.

In case of an emergency, if you *absolutely must* lift something heavier than what you're permitted, at least wear your abdominal binder for support. If you find yourself straining or becoming weak, do not lift the item under any circumstances.

Deep-Breathing and Leg-Pumping Exercises

As far as exercising goes, it's important to continue pretty much the same regimen you followed while in the hospital. This includes getting up and walking around each hour that you are awake. Also don't forget to use your incentive spirometer every hour during waking hours. At other times, continue to breathe deeply. Also, do your leg-pumping exercises as often as you think about it—at least a thousand times a day. Remember to keep your legs elevated when lying or sitting and don't cross them. This is important since, for about six weeks following surgery, you are still at risk for developing pneumonia or a blood clot. Once you've regained your strength, you'll be adding other exercises to your routine. This is discussed later in this chapter.

Clothing

Remember to wear only loose-fitting clothing for the first five to six weeks following surgery to give your surgical incision a chance to heal completely. Anything that causes friction, even a small amount, around your abdomen can damage your wound and cause it to open or become infected. Therefore, avoid wearing anything with an elastic waistband or anything that is constricting around the abdomen. Especially when wearing your abdominal binder, be sure to protect your wound by keeping the dressings on or by wearing a soft undergarment below the binder.

Later, after you've healed from your surgery and begin to lose weight, you'll be dropping sizes. Wait until you've reached your target weight before buying a whole new wardrobe. Instead, buy or borrow a few pieces of versatile clothing. Secondhand shops are a great place to find bargains on clothing you'll be wearing only temporarily. Also, support groups often have clothing swaps. Group members often share clothing that is almost like new since it was worn for only a short time. With your rapid weight loss, you too will be wearing much of this "new" clothing for a very brief time. Swapping clothing is a wonderful way to share with your support group friends. If your support group doesn't have a clothing swap in place, you may want to organize one.

Keeping an Eye on Your Surgical Wound

In about one in three cases following open surgery, and less frequently following laparoscopic surgery, pinkish watery fluid will drain from the surgical wound. This may last for a few days or up to seven days. This drainage is normal. However, if you notice that your wound, or part of it, is becoming inflamed as indicated by pain, redness, and/or swelling, call your surgeon and make an appointment to see him within a day or two. He will likely take a culture to check for a bacterial infection and start you on antibiotics if necessary. Thereafter, the wound will be observed periodically to make sure it's healing. In a small percentage of cases in which an infection develops, the wound will need to be opened and packed. If so, this may take several weeks to heal since the wound is usually quite deep. Eventually, the fat layer will turn a pinkish to salmon color, and the wound can then be taped or sewn together, with or without some small drains.

Dealing with the Gastrostomy Tube (G-Tube)

If you had a gastrostomy tube inserted during surgery, it will be removed at your first or second visit to the surgeon's office. If, however, you have some difficulty consuming enough fluids or food, it may be used to provide your body with adequate fluids for a while. Usually, you—or someone helping you—will draw up a specified number of ounces of fluid in a large syringe and will inject it into the tube. Your medicines, liquid or liquefied, can also be given through this tube if necessary. Before discharge, the hospital nursing staff will instruct you on how to accomplish this relatively easy task.

Managing Pain

For your first few days at home, you may choose to take the pain medication your surgeon prescribed. (If you need the medication, we recommend that you crush or liquefy it and add it to your liquids or purées.) However, your need for pain medication specifically for abdominal pain should be very little or absent within a few days after your discharge from the hospital. If the pain does not subside or if it begins to get worse, call your surgeon. Be aware that pain in your abdomen can be the result of a muscle tear. This can happen especially if you do not have abdominal support while lifting. This pain, which is usually moderate, can last for weeks or months. It will usually be located in a small area on your abdomen and may be felt only when you move or press on that area. To be sure that this pain is nothing more serious, it is wise to have your surgeon examine you.

Driving and Traveling After Surgery

We recommend that you avoid driving for at least two weeks following your surgery. Then, for the next several weeks, drive only if there is an urgent need to do so and only for short distances—that is, less than five minutes of driving time. Remember, while you're sitting, you need to have your legs up to avoid blood clots and swelling. You can't possibly do this if you're driving. That's why you should drive *only* if there is an absolute and urgent need.

Also, long-distance travel for the first few months following surgery is probably more stress than your recovering body should be subjected to. Therefore, avoid traveling unless it's for a very good reason. Moreover, the further you go, the further away from your surgeon's office you will be. You'll want to be as close as possible to the office in case of an emergency.

Engaging in Sexual Activity

There is no limitation on your sexual activity during recovery unless your common sense suggests otherwise. Largely due to hormonal changes, sex drive is often increased in the majority of people following their massive weight loss. If you are a woman, be sure to use birth control to avoid pregnancy. See the inset "Wait to Become Pregnant" on page 160.

Keeping an Eye Out for Depression

In our experience, 25 to 30 percent of patients become depressed following weight-loss surgery. Since it is hard to predict who will become depressed and who won't, anyone who has the surgery needs to be aware of the possibility that some level of depression may develop.

For a period of time after surgery, you may experience depression due to the effects of the anesthesia you received during the procedure. Also, and more important, after surgery, your brain will be undergoing changes in its chemistry, since smaller amounts of nutrients are being absorbed into your semi-fasting body. As a result of these nutritional changes, your body may produce less serotonin—a chemical in your brain and nerves associated with pleasure. Low levels of serotonin have been linked to depression. This

Wait to Become Pregnant

Morbidly obese women frequently have problems becoming pregnant due to irregular menstrual cycles. In cases where infertility is not a problem, pregnancy in an obese woman may be high risk due to factors such as hypertension and diabetes. There may be an increased risk for spontaneous abortion, preeclampsia, Cesarean section, and a slightly increased risk of deep venous thrombosis. This can be a frightening prognosis. Therefore, the question on many a woman's mind is, "After my surgery, will I be able to get pregnant and have a safe pregnancy?" In most cases, once your weight has leveled off and your body has healed and your comorbidities have improved, the answer is yes. However, it's wise to avoid becoming pregnant for at least a year and a half to two years after surgery. Pregnancy robs your body of nutrients to feed your growing fetus, nutrients you so desperately need during your period of massive weight loss. Also, you may not be able to provide the fetus with enough nutrients for its proper development. In addition, pregnancy during this period can, understandably, decrease the amount of weight you'll lose.

Because many women were unsuccessful in their efforts to conceive before they had the surgery, they may not think it's necessary to use birth control. However, weight loss can enormously increase a woman's chance of becoming pregnant, so past difficulty is no indication or guarantee of a lack of fertility. We strongly recommend the use of birth control to prevent pregnancy until your weight completely levels off. It's best to give yourself an additional three months at your new weight. Be sure to speak to your surgeon about the best form of contraception for you.

form of depression may persist for as long as it takes for your weight loss to level off completely. It can become serious and needs to be treated.

Moreover, weight-loss surgery is a tool that can very effectively change your body but not your mind. Preexisting depression, which is common in many of our patients, will not automatically disappear. In addition, in some people, the very stressors that caused weight gain and the issues of weight prejudice and abuse that may have existed will also not disappear after surgery. Food can no longer be used to handle these feelings or to "numb out." As a result, when one returns home, these feelings may return with a vengeance, creating increased depression.

In addition, the dramatic change in appearance that results from weight loss may have consequences you did not foresee. Some people may find the

When your weight has stabilized, your surgeon will probably be glad to welcome another member into his extended family. Since you will be at an increased risk for anemia during pregnancy—especially if you've had gastric bypass of any type—your doctor may have a list of precautions for you to follow along with the recommendation to take additional vitamins, including folic acid and vitamin B_{12}, as well as iron. In fact, as soon as you become aware of your pregnancy, see a nutritionist to determine your baseline nutritional status. Laboratory results can help your nutritionist and other health-care professionals determine the proper adjustments early on. Continuing to see a nutritionist, as well as other health-care professionals, each month during your pregnancy is important.

Pregnancy is not the time to maintain a strict diet. If you do not gain weight during pregnancy, your baby can run the risk of intrauterine growth retardation, fetal abnormality, or low birth weight. These can be serious problems. This is also not the time to abandon compliance with your program. Moderation is the key. Some doctors suggest a weight gain of about 26 pounds as optimal, although this varies widely. Again, remain closely monitored and don't be afraid to ask questions.

With that said, be aware that some of our patients have become pregnant within the first year of their surgery despite our precautions. Fortunately, they and their babies were fine with proper care. If you should become pregnant during your weight-loss period, call your surgeon's office right away for an appointment. He and your obstetrician will follow your pregnancy closely to help ensure success.

"changed you" difficult to get used to. As a result, some relationships will change, and some may even be lost. In fact, so many aspects of your life will be changing that you may find the effects quite dizzying. All of this and the speed at which it happens can, at times, prove depressing. Again, food will not be available to create artificial calm or ease the pain.

In these cases, professional counseling can provide a necessary supportive outlet and can help to resolve old issues, relieve present stressors, deal with the multiple and rapid changes taking place, and help you to look forward to a clearer and brighter future. As you continue to read, you may also find that knowing you are not alone can help ease the burdensome and sometimes complicated feelings you are experiencing.

The symptoms of depression were discussed in Chapter 8 on page 145.

Review them and think seriously about whether or not you are experiencing any of the symptoms. If so, contact your surgeon and your health-care practitioner as soon as possible. All psychological consultations are kept strictly confidential. It's better to seek help early on before you become seriously depressed—and remember, depression is *not* your fault—it is likely a product of the chemical changes your body is undergoing.

Although it's not always the case, treatment for depression may include a mild, non-habit-forming antidepressant or an adjustment to an antidepressant medication you may already be taking. If your surgeon decides that antidepressants are right for your case, it's a good idea to stay on the medication at least until your weight loss levels off completely, or until your surgeon says otherwise. Do *not* stop taking your medication without discussing it with your doctor.

Avoiding Certain Medications

Drugs commonly used for the treatment of arthritis, bursitis, tendonitis, and for back pain can irritate your stomach lining, which could develop into a bleeding ulcer. For this reason, you need to be aware of which drugs to avoid and which are safe to take—in moderation, of course. Use the following as a guide, and be sure to ask your surgeon for a list of approved medications.

Drugs to Avoid

- Advil
- alcohol
- Aleve
- Alka-Seltzer
- Ascriptin
- aspirin
- Bufferin
- Coricidin
- cortisone
- Dolobid
- Empirin
- Excedrin
- Feldene
- fiorinal
- ibuprofen
- Indocin
- Meclomen
- Motrin
- Nalfon
- Naprosyn
- Norgesic
- Pepto-Bismol
- Tolectin
- Vanquish

Drugs You Can Safely Take in Moderation

- acetaminophen
- Anacin-3
- Datril
- Fioricet
- Panadol
- Tylenol

Don't forget that for the first five to six weeks after your surgery, your medication *must* be liquefied or crushed and added to liquids or purées. Also, don't take all your medications at once. Take them with sips of water and then wait at least a few minutes to avoid their gumming up in or clogging your stomach pouch, which can cause pain or feedback.

Avoiding Blood Donations

People who have had weight-loss surgery often have a difficult time getting or absorbing enough iron, vitamins, and other nutrients from their food to enable their bodies to produce enough hemoglobin—the oxygen-carrying portion of the red blood cell. Because of this, they are at risk for anemia. Therefore, as a rule, we recommend that our patients avoid donating blood for life.

Returning to Work

If you're like most weight-loss surgery patients, you should be able to return to work within four to six weeks. If you underwent laparoscopic surgery, you may be able to return to work even sooner than this, perhaps within two to four weeks. That's fine, of course, if your job isn't physically demanding. If it is, you may want to take a few additional weeks to recover. In some cases, people will return to work on a part-time basis until they feel strong enough for full-time work. Be sure to decide what's best for you, and don't return to work sooner than you feel capable of resuming your work-related activities.

EMERGENCIES

If you have a medical or surgical emergency, you might be tempted to just call your regular doctor. This is not a good idea. You must call your surgeon's office. Since weight-loss surgery is a relatively new area of specialty, you cannot expect your family doctor to be familiar with the important details of how to manage your problems, many of which are unique to the surgery. Your surgeon knows you inside and out, so be sure to rely upon him.

Speak with your surgeon directly or ask a support person who is with you to explain your problems to the surgeon. Because patients are being discharged earlier from the hospital, complications that may have been picked up during your hospital stay may not be caught. If you suspect that you've developed a complication, you must report it to your surgeon right away.

Depending on what you describe, your surgeon may instruct you to go to the emergency room or to make a visit to his office.

Although you are aware of what type of things can go wrong—such as leaks, bleeding, diarrhea, nausea, vomiting, infection, high temperature, increased heart rate or breathing, blood clots, dizziness, and depression—you are not expected to make a self-diagnosis. It is your surgeon's job to diagnose the problem. However, you should be aware of the warning signs of a serious problem for which you must seek help. Some of these are listed below. Be sure to call your surgeon if any of the following occurs:

- Your temperature is 101°F or higher.

- Your resting heart rate is 110 to 120 beats per minute.

- You have difficulty breathing or experience rapid breathing—twenty-five to thirty breaths or more per minute.

- The swelling in your legs has increased, especially if just on one side.

- You experience chest pain (this is different from pain in the midline of your upper abdomen, which is likely related to the surgery).

- Your skin has lost color and becomes pale.

- You feel weak and very tired and do not want to or cannot muster the strength to move.

- You feel sad or irritable and have no desire to get up or do anything all day.

- You're suffering from insomnia, and you feel sleepy most or all of the time.

- You are confused and "not talking right"—that is, you're making little sense when you speak or you are slurring your words.

- You are vomiting everything you swallow or cannot keep any clear liquids down for a day or more.

- You are vomiting blood.

- Your stool contains blood.

- You are shaking and have the chills.

- You have increased pain in your wound that pain medicine doesn't help.

- Your wound or drain site is oozing pus, green fluid, stool, or recently eaten food.

- A very large or increased amount of fluid is draining from your wound.

- You experience severe diarrhea that doesn't let up.

- You have a protruding bulge, perhaps a hernia, that you may not be able to push back in place. (For more information about hernias, see the inset "About Ventral Hernias" below.)

- You have severe cramping abdominal pain with or without a swollen abdomen.

- You have severe steady abdominal pain that does not seem to be getting any better.

If you cannot reach your surgeon, go to the emergency room of the nearest hopital. If you do need to go to the hospital, you'll want to bring

About Ventral Hernias

A hernia is an abnormal protrusion of an organ or other body tissue through an opening in your body wall or internal tissues. The incision in your abdomen is very deep. Part of it may become stretched so far that an opening in your abdominal wall occurs. Fat, some of the intestines, or other abdominal content may push out into this opening. This is called a *ventral hernia*.

If you have a ventral hernia, you may notice a bulge in your incision. In some cases, when you cough or strain, you may actually feel something pushing out of a defect or hole in your incision or elsewhere in your abdominal wall. Be sure to call your surgeon if you notice anything like this as soon as it occurs. You may be able to wait to have the ventral hernia repaired, although it does tend to cause some pain. Your surgeon will advise you whether or not it is wise to wait; don't try to make this determination for yourself. In most cases, if part of your intestines becomes stuck inside the hernia, it is a medical emergency. The health of your intestines is at risk. If you are unable to push the bulge back into your abdomen while on your back and relaxing the abdominal muscles, go to the emergency room and have them call your surgeon. You may need emergency surgery.

To prevent a ventral hernia from developing, wear your abdominal binder regularly and do not lift more than 25 pounds or similarly strain your abdomen for six months after your surgery.

along an emergency notice card, or Med-Alert card. This card, which is usually provided by your surgeon, certifies that you've had bariatric surgery and sometimes provides a diagram of the procedure. (If you surgeon does not provide such a card, ask for one.) Be sure to keep the card in your wallet for easy access. Also, be sure to insist that the emergency-room physician call your surgeon to discuss the complication that you are experiencing.

ASSESSING YOUR WEIGHT-LOSS PROGRESS

When you get home, you'll naturally want to weigh yourself. If you do, don't be surprised if you weigh more, not less, than you did before surgery. This extra weight is due to fluid retention—your body will likely hold on to much of the fluid that was pumped into it during your stay at the hospital. For a while, this fluid retention will continue to a greater or lesser degree. If you weigh yourself daily, you'll see that your weight, like the stock market, can be unpredictable, confusing, and perhaps demoralizing. It's best to choose one day a week to weigh yourself, and do it first thing in the morning. This is better for morale and won't hang you up with worries about the frequent "ups and downs" of the scale, which really have little meaning. The changes in your body are more reliable indicators of how you're doing. You'll know how you are doing when you feel better, stronger, and more able to get around. Rest assured, your weight will decrease, but it will take time.

Hopefully, you've taken the advice in Chapter 7 to take your picture and record your measurements in a notebook. From time to time, take your measurements again and compare the numbers. If you choose, you can also record your weight and clothing sizes for comparison. Chances are you'll see that you are losing inches even if the numbers on your scale are not dropping. Also, it's important to keep in mind that, if you are engaging in resistance training, you are building muscle while shedding fat. Muscle weighs more than fat, so the pounds on the scale may not be dropping as much as you would expect. The best way to determine your progress is really by sight and feel.

Weight is not lost in a steady decline. Rather, some weight is lost, and then it levels off. Then, it goes down again. This occurs partly because fat breaks down into carbon dioxide and water. The carbon dioxide is breathed out and the water is removed from your body mostly through urine, stools, and sweat. Sometimes, though, your body will hold on to the water, and though fat has been lost, your weight remains the same. You'll eventually lose the extra water, but this will occur in spurts rather than steadily. This is why the typical weight-loss pattern following surgery is described as a series of plateaus in which you lose weight, level off, lose weight, and so on.

Plateaus and all, the overall effect is still exciting. It's not unusual for you to lose about 10 percent of your weight in the first six or so weeks following surgery. For example, if you were 270 pounds at the time of your surgery, you will lose about 27 pounds those first six or so weeks. People who have been fitted with inflatable bands will lose weight a little more slowly, depending upon how often and how much the band is adjusted. Typically, their weight loss will be less dramatic, but it will continue for about three years as opposed to twelve to twenty-four months following gastroplasty, gastric bypass, and related types of weight-loss procedures. In any event, most weight-loss-surgery patients lose anywhere from 10 to 20 pounds by the time their skin sutures or staples are removed. Thereafter, the average weight loss can be about 10 pounds per month until close to one-third of the starting weight has been lost.

Everyone's "window of opportunity" is different. Generally speaking, the weight-loss period can start tapering off around nine months, especially in the case of shorter women. People who exercise regularly can keep this window open for as long as two years. The more active you are, the more muscle you will develop. When you have more muscle available for burning calories, your metabolism will speed up and burn more of your fat. (See the section "Your New Exercise Program" on page 174.)

Try not to be distressed or frustrated by "how long it takes" to lose weight. After all, you didn't put your weight on overnight, and you knew going in that this process takes time. When you find yourself getting impatient, ask yourself, "When did I ever regularly lose ten pounds or so per month?" The answer will probably be "never." Take pleasure in the pounds you lose and your ever-changing body. Remember to help your body in its weight-loss efforts by eating properly and exercising regularly. You'll find some helpful advice about this in the following sections.

YOUR NEW EATING PLAN

In most cases, for the first six months or so after surgery, the new stomach pouch or gastric band limits the amount of calories you can consume to about 500 to 800 calories a day. Sooner or later, however, the amount of food that can be comfortably eaten at one time will increase. When you can eat more, do not exceed 1,200 calories daily if you are a woman and no more than 1,500 calories if you are a man. Usually, this higher-calorie intake will reduce the amount of weight you lose or, later on, may even result in your regaining some of the weight. Therefore, it is critical that you immediately and completely change your eating habits by consuming only three or four small meals each day and drinking low-calorie beverages between meals to help keep you full and hydrated. You will need to avoid snacking between your meals unless you are told to take extra protein to meet your protein needs.

Let's take a look at the importance of eating properly and what your body needs to keep you strong and healthy during your weight loss.

Changing Your Eating Habits

During presurgery discussions, many of our patients talk about their habit of eating large amounts of food very quickly, often gulping it down without chewing properly. After weight-loss surgery, such eating habits are obviously no longer possible. Eating too quickly, as well as eating certain foods, can cause feedback (see the inset "A Message From Your Stomach" on page 169).

During the first few weeks following your surgery, you'll feel full after as little as 2 to 3 ounces of liquids or purées. You may notice this "full" feeling in your upper abdomen quite clearly, or feel a slightly uncomfortable sensation or tightness behind the lower end of your breastbone. Once you have learned what "full" feels like, watch for it at each meal. As soon as you experience that "full" feeling, stop eating. If you do not stop eating when your body signals you to stop, you may stuff your stomach pouch so full that it will cause pain in your upper abdomen, and perhaps in your back. You may also become nauseated with or without vomiting. Later, bad habbits like this can cause you to regain the lost weight.

Daily Fluid Intake

Adequate fluid intake is a must to keep you from becoming dehydrated and fatigued. After surgery, you must drink approximately 64 ounces of fluid each day, over the course of the day in small amounts. Sip, sip, sip is the key. Most of us are accustomed to gulping large amounts of liquid. This is no longer possible. Some people like to use "sippy" cups—the small lidded spill-proof cups with a spout often used by toddlers. If you decide to go this route, enjoy this "return to childhood" and make it fun. You might want to get a sippy cup in your favorite color and keep it close at hand.

It's important to measure the amount of fluid you're drinking. Often-

A Message From Your Stomach

Feedback—the slight regurgitation of food; that is, the food goes down and then comes back up—is a message from your stomach pouch telling you to take smaller bites, sip your beverages more slowly, chew your food more thoroughly, and/or pause longer between taking bites and/or sips. Feedback is not the same thing as vomiting due to an illness. Rather, it is a signal from your body that you need to change your eating or drinking behavior. Since feedback is unpleasant, you'll want to "listen" carefully for your stomach's messages and take them seriously.

While some weight-loss-surgery patients claim to have never experienced it, most people do get a little feedback. Anytime you experience it, try to figure out what caused it. Did you eat or drink too quickly? Did you eat or drink too much? Did a certain food have this effect? (By the way, rice, especially sticky or clumpy; bread; and red meat are three common offenders.)

Once you've figured out what caused your feedback, make a note of it. Then, avoid repeating that behavior or eating that food at any of your meals. At some later time, you may be able to try the offending foods again, in small amounts to start with, but you will always need to eat and drink slowly and chew thoroughly. In Chapter 8, we discussed smaller-sized dinnerware—small cups, straws, spoons, and "sippy" cups. Using these items can help you to prevent feedback by limiting the amount of food you can take in at one time.

times, people think they're drinking enough, but when they begin measuring, they discover they aren't coming near the 64-ounce mark. So, be sure to keep close track.

Before surgery, you may have been accustomed to drinking beverages with your meals, as many of us are. After surgery, this is not permitted. If you fill your stomach pouch with liquid at mealtimes, there will be no room for protein and the other basic nutrients your body needs to avoid malnutrition. Also, drinking at mealtimes can result in the stacking of solids and liquids in your stomach pouch, which can lead to nausea, vomiting, or discomfort. Moreover, drinking soon after your meal can "wash out" the food in your stomach pouch and may make you feel less full. Therefore, drink only between meals. Some surgeons recommend not drinking for the thirty to sixty minutes leading up to mealtimes and waiting for the same amount of time to pass after mealtimes before drinking.

So, what types of beverages should you drink? There are many choices, but water is at the top of the list. If your tap water is unsafe or doesn't taste good, consider purchasing bottled water or bottles with water filters, or getting a water cooler for your home. If you choose a water cooler that also provides hot water, it'll be a lot easier to prepare herbal tea or broth. With cold and hot water on hand at the touch of a button, you may be more likely to drink more often.

Other acceptable beverages include skim milk, decaffeinated coffee or tea, fruit juices diluted with water (at least fifty-fifty), and sugar-free drink mixes, which come in a wide variety of flavors. Herbal teas, which are naturally decaffeinated, are also a good option. If you've never been a big herbal tea drinker, purchase an herbal tea variety pack to discover which flavors you like best. Maintaining a large fluid intake can be difficult, but it is absolutely essential for long-term compliance and overall health. Variety is often key. Discover which drinks you like best, and keep a varied supply on hand.

Cautions About Fluid Intake

Be sure to read labels so that you are thoroughly familiar with the contents of any beverage or beverage mix you are thinking about purchasing. Key words to be on the lookout for include "carbonated water," "high-fructose corn syrup" (or any other form of added sugar), and "caffeine." Put down anything that contains these items for the reasons explained below. Also, avoid high-calorie beverages, which can hinder your weight-loss efforts.

Carbonated beverages can distend or stretch the stomach pouch and its connection with your intestines. Therefore, if you were used to drinking soda, diet or otherwise, we highly recommend that you no longer drink it to avoid damaging your pouch.

Also, avoid drinking beverages with added sugar. They are high in empty calories and will cause an immediate increase in your blood sugar levels, possibly causing discomfort and dumping syndrome (see page 48).

Moreover, avoid all caffeine-containing drinks, including tea and coffee, since caffeine can impede postsurgical success. Caffeine can cause ulcers, damage the stomach lining, contribute to calcium loss, and raise blood pressure and heart rate. Caffeine can also raise stress levels and become a cause of high-carbohydrate, stress-related eating.

Also be wary of alcohol consumption for several reasons. First of all, alcohol is high in calories, nutritionally void, and tends to blunt weight loss. Also, after surgery, alcohol is more quickly absorbed by the body and can have disastrous results. You can become intoxicated from small amounts of alcohol much more easily. (By all means, if you do have even one drink, *do not* drive, since you don't know what effect this will have on you.) Furthermore, people who have had gastric bypass surgery are more prone to liver damage as a result of alcohol consumption. It's best to avoid consuming alcohol.

Also, keep in mind that some over-the-counter medications contain high levels of alcohol. Some contain caffeine. Once again, read all labels to make sure you're not taking anything in that will have a negative effect on your health and recovery.

Protein Intake

In addition to taking in adequate fluids, you will need to consume 60 to 80 grams of protein each day. At first, getting this much protein will take a lot of attention and effort on your part. You may need to keep written track of your protein intake to make sure you're getting enough to keep your body nourished and healthy.

To meet your daily protein needs, you'll need to eat mostly protein-rich foods, such as fish, eggs, poultry, beef, dairy, and protein supplements. At mealtimes, be sure to eat your protein-rich foods first so that you don't fill up on non-protein-rich items. Therefore, you must be very picky and careful when choosing your foods to make sure you include high-protein ones at each meal.

Once again, you'll need to keep close track of how many grams you consume each day. To help, Table 9.1 on page 172 lists the approximate protein content of some common foods and drinks used postsurgically.

There's a good chance you'll need to take a protein supplement every day for months, or even years, to meet your daily protein needs. If so, you'll surgeon and nutritionist will let you know. We often recommend ProMod or UNJURY (three scoops daily) to our patients. However, there are dozens of protein supplements on the market, and your surgeon will be able to provide you with a list of them. Your surgeon or doctor will most likely monitor your protein status from time to time and will let you know if you need to adjust your dosage of protein supplements. Be sure to ask about your protein status if your doctor doesn't mention it. Do not stop taking your protein supplement on your own. If you think you're getting enough protein from your diet, keep a diet diary listing everything you eat and drink for at least seven days and show it to your doctor. He will help you determine if you're taking in adequate amounts of protein without supplements.

TABLE 9.1 PROTEIN CONTENT OF COMMON POSTSURGICAL FOODS AND DRINKS

FOOD (PURÉE OR LIQUID)	SERVING SIZE	PROTEIN CONTENT*
Applesauce	1 ounce	0.05 g
Banana	1 medium	1.0 g
Beans (cooked and/or refried)	1 ounce	1.5–2.0 g
Buttermilk	1 ounce	1.0 g
Celery (raw)	1 stalk	0.3 g
Cottage cheese	1 ounce	3.5 g
Crabmeat, imitation	1 ounce	1.5–2.0 g
Cream of Wheat	$\frac{1}{2}$ cup	1.85 g
Egg	1 medium	5.5 g
Fish	1 ounce	6–8 g
Frankfurter (chicken, veggie, or soy)	1 frank	5–9 g
Grapes	1 ounce	0.1 g
Milk	1 ounce	2.0 g
Oatmeal	1 ounce	0.75 g
Orange	1 medium	1 g
Poultry (skinless)	1 ounce	6–8 g
Protein supplement powder (specifically, ProMod Protein Supplement powder)	1 scoop	5.0 g
Raisins	1 ounce	1.25 g
Shrimp	1 ounce	7.0 g
Tangerine	1 medium	1.0 g
Vegetables (canned)	1 ounce	0.25 g
Vegetables (fresh, cooked)	1 ounce	0.40–0.75 g
Veggie burger	1 pattie	5.5 g
Vitamite 100, Non-Dairy Beverage	1 serving	0.10 g
Yogurt	1 ounce	1.0 g

*All values are approximate and may vary by type and brand.

Foods to Avoid

Avoid high-calorie, sugar-rich foods such as candy, jams, and jelly. (Be sure to avoid products made with brown sugar as well as white sugar.) Also avoid fat-laden foods, including fried foods and ice cream. Other foods to avoid include honey, mayonnaise, oil, butter, margarine, cream, gravies, sauces, and salad dressings. These foods provide a lot of hollow, useless calories without providing much nutritional value. Therefore, you must make a serious effort to avoid consuming them in any quantity. The price you'll pay for consuming them will be less of a weight loss than you're hoping for.

For at least six months, you should also avoid eating red meat, bread, and rice (brown and white), as well as high-fiber foods, since they are more difficult to digest.

Nutritional Supplements

Your nutritional intake and absorption have been purposely limited by weight-loss surgery. Therefore, you will need to make up for this by taking nutritional supplements—a multivitamin with iron and, later, a separate calcium supplement.

Usually you'll be instructed to start supplementing right away by taking one chewable multivitamin with iron before breakfast, lunch, and dinner daily. Take it with some orange, grapefruit, or other citrus juice. Don't take it with food, other medications, supplements, cocoa, tea, coffee, or diet sodas—they interfere with the absorption of iron.

At first, children's chewable multivitamins with iron are a good option since they are easily crushed and swallowed, and usually taste good. Later, in about six to ten weeks, you should be able to handle adult vitamins without any problem. At that point, you may be instructed to take two supplements each day with a half cup of diluted citrus juice.

A Weight-Loss Pitfall

When the surgical swelling has gone down and you have gotten used to your new anatomy, you will find that you can nibble on food or drink high-calorie beverages all day long without too much discomfort. Nibbling like this and drinking high-calorie beverages instead of water or other acceptable drinks are self-destructive. This behavior will prevent you from losing weight, and you've been through far too much to hinder your efforts now.

Calcium is needed by your body to prevent calcium deficiency as a result of surgery. Also, calcium supplementation together with regular exercise will help you prevent osteoporosis in later years. You'll need about 1,500 mg of elemental calcium daily. Check with your nutritionist about when you should start taking calcium supplements. He may advise you to wait a month or so until you are able to swallow pills more easily or may recommend a chewable form of calcium.

When you do take a calcium supplement, be sure to take it at least a half hour apart from your multivitamin with iron. Calcium, being an alkali (the opposite of acidic), interferes with iron absorption, which needs an acidic environment to be absorbed.

Tums antacids are a good source of chewable calcium. Depending on the strength of the product, you'll need to take about three to seven tablets to meet your supplemental calcium quota. You can also get about the same amount of calcium by taking a product such as Caltrate 600 (three tablets) or Calel-D (three tablets) or by taking one heaping teaspoon of calcium carbonate powder or the appropriate amount of other preparations such as calcium citrate at bedtime. Find a calcium product that you like with the help of your nutritionist and be sure to take it daily.

Special Meal Cards

Some surgeons provide "restaurant cards" or "eating out cards" that certify that you have had your stomach surgically reduced in size and request that you be charged for a smaller portion, be able to share with a companion, or be allowed to order from the less-expensive children's menu. Many restaurants honor these cards. If your surgeon does not provide a meal card, ask for one. Keep the card in your wallet or purse, so it's handy when you need to present it to the management at a restaurant you're visiting.

YOUR NEW EXERCISE PROGRAM

Weight-loss surgery is only a tool, a tool you'll need to make work for you. People who make the best progress are those who work hard at their weight-loss program, which includes regular exercise. Don't cheat yourself out of this important aspect of weight loss. You'll want your body to have every advantage to make your goals a reality. The more you weigh, the harder it is to reach your goal weight. Therefore, exercise *must* become part of your lifestyle. Not only does it help you achieve your weight-loss

An Overview of Basic Nutrition Principles

The instructions you receive concerning dietary matters may vary somewhat from surgeon to surgeon and case by case. There are, however, some basic nutrition principles that most surgeons agree upon. These are listed below. As always, if your surgeon's recommendations differ from these, follow your surgeon's instructions.

- **Start your solid diet with easy-to-chew foods.**
When you are permitted to eat solid foods, start with soft, easy-to-chew foods such as mashed potatoes and steamed vegetables. Chew these foods thoroughly (about twenty bites per mouthful) until they are practically liquefied before swallowing them.

- **Eat slowly, and stop eating as soon as you begin to feel full.**
Gulping down your food can cause serious problems, such as extreme discomfort. Eating too quickly and too much can also stretch out your stomach pouch and greatly hinder your weight-loss efforts. You need to eat your food slowly and chew it thoroughly. Pay very close attention to your body's signal that you have had enough.

- **Do not drink beverages with your meals.**
Stop drinking at least a half hour before each meal. Wait another half hour after meals to begin sipping your beverage again. (See the section "Daily Fluid Intake" on page 168.)

- **Introduce new foods into your diet one at a time.**
It's important to add only one new food into your diet at a time, since trying more than one new type of food will make it difficult to identify an offending food if problems arise. When adding the new food, experiment with a very small amount. If it doesn't cause any problem, you can slightly increase the amount you eat on a different day to see if it still goes down okay in a larger amount.

- **Take all of your nutritional supplements as directed.**
When a diet provides fewer than 1,200 calories daily, it is unlikely that your body's nutritional needs can be met without supplementation. In the absence of the proper nutrients, you can develop osteoporosis or certain nutrient deficiencies. Therefore, be sure to take all supplements as directed.

You can put yourself at risk by making unapproved substitutions or discontinuing supplementation on your own, so speak with your nutritionist about any changes you think are necessary.

- **Drink at least 64 ounces of acceptable fluids each day.**
Sip approved beverages throughout the day from a small cup to prevent gulping. Stop drinking for at least a half hour before and after meals. Keep written track of how much fluid you take in to avoid drinking too little.

- **Take in at least 60 to 80 grams of protein daily.**
Follow your surgeon's and nutritionist's advice regarding protein consumption. If this includes taking supplemental protein, be sure to comply. During the period of weight loss, getting adequate protein is absolutely essential for good health.

- **Eat three or four small meals each day without snacking or skipping meals.**
Schedule your mealtimes and eat at approximately the same times each day. Don't skip meals since your body depends on the nutrients you take in during those times. Avoid snacking between meals, as this will surely interfere with your weight-loss efforts.

- **Avoid hollow-calorie foods and beverages.**
Alcohol, soda, fat-laden foods, sugar-rich snacks and candies, fried foods, and other unhealthy foods and beverages all interfere with your weight-loss efforts and general health. Moreover, consuming them in place of protein-rich foods will put you at risk for a protein deficiency. If you wish for something "sweet" now and again, use artificial sweeteners such as NutraSweet (aspartame), Sweet'N Low (saccharin), or Splenda (sucralose).

- **Regular follow-up with a nutritionist is essential.**
Be sure to maintain your relationship with a nutritionist for the rest of your life. If any dietary problems develop or if you have any questions concerning any nutritional matters between appointments, be sure to call your nutritionist to discuss them. Your surgeon can also provide some helpful information should the need arise. Of course, your follow-ups are not limited to your nutritionist. You will also need to get regular checkups from your regular doctor and your surgeon for the rest of your life.

goals quicker, it also helps maintain bone density, aids in weight-loss maintenance, increases strength and balance, boosts your energy levels, lifts your mood, and improves the overall quality of life. In some cases, exercise can help reduce sagging skin, but its ability to shrink back the skin depends on many factors. (There's more on concerns about sagging skin in Chapter 10.)

During exercise, the feel-good chemicals known as *endorphins* are released in the brain, providing a natural sense of well-being. You can become "addicted" to this feeling, which you'll find yourself missing if you skip exercise. That's a good thing. The more you exercise, the more you'll look forward to your next session.

There are two types of exercise—aerobic (with oxygen) and anaerobic (without oxygen). Aerobic exercise includes activities such as walking, running, jogging, or swimming, and anaerobic exercises include activities such as resistance training and weight lifting. In the beginning, walking will be your best choice. As you already know, it's very import to get up and walk around several times a day after your surgery. As your strength increases, extend the distance or length of time that you walk. Don't walk just to get around; walk enough so that it eventually becomes a weight-loss exercise. Even after you lose your weight, make walking for exercise a regular habit to keep you in good shape and to maintain your weight loss.

The recommended walking distance after surgery is about 100 yards. If you have a problem walking, walk only about 50 to 70 percent of your maximum distance. After a week or so, increase your walking distance by about one-third and keep increasing it. A realistic goal is to reach one mile twice a day at the end of your first month with a longer-term goal of at least two miles twice a day. If you cannot reach this goal, just do the best you can.

As you become stronger, you'll want to expand your repertoire of exercises. While shedding fat, you need to conserve and build up your body's muscle mass. Muscle helps your body burn additional calories, increases your strength, and boosts your energy levels. These are all essential elements in your lifelong weight-loss program. This is where resistance training and/or lifting weights are beneficial.

When developing an exercise program, safety should be first and foremost on your mind. Enjoyment is also an important aspect of any exercise program. We've asked our colleague Barbara Metcalf, R.N., the program director of Pacific Laparoscopy in San Francisco, to provide us with some guidelines for developing a safe and effective exercise program. Ms. Metcalf is a nationally recognized authority on exercise for those who have had weight-loss surgery, so her input is very much appreciated. We've adapted her ideas and have incorporated them into the following pointers.

- Speak with your doctor about your exercise plan *before* you start your program to get his okay.

- Consult a fitness expert, such as a personal trainer, or read a few books on fitness to learn about the various exercises available to you, how to do them properly, and what muscles they work.

- *Do not* do any abdominal exercises, such as crunches, until your surgeon has cleared you to do so. Depending on the type of surgery you've had, this may be around the eight- to twelve-week mark. When you do start to work on your abs, be sure to perform the exercise properly to avoid injury. (See the inset "Abdominal Crunches" below.)

- Always warm up before exercise and cool down after exercise by stretching for a few minutes at least. This will help you avoid injuries. It also improves joint flexibility and loosens tight muscles. Stretching strengthens your tendons and feels really good, especially when your muscles are warmed up from exercise. Enjoy that stretching!

- Use the right equipment. For example, make sure your shoes fit well and provide good support.

- Use safety devices, such as helmets, goggles, and gloves, when necessary.

- Use common sense, be patient, and have fun!

Abdominal Crunches

When you've been cleared by your doctor to start doing abdominal crunches, pay close attention to your body's signals. Start slowly and increase your repetitions gradually. It's important to do crunches properly so that you don't strain your neck. Lie on your back with your knees bent at about a 90-degree angle. Clasp your hands behind your head with your elbows flat on the floor. (If you can see your elbows, your arms are not in the proper position.) Lift your head and arms a few inches off the floor and then lower yourself back to the floor; feel the muscles in your abdomen working. Start with about ten repetitions. As you progress and your abs begin to strengthen, you'll be able to increase your repetitions for maximum benefit.

- Listen to your body; if something hurts, don't do it!

- Choose activities that are going to work for you. Visualize what you'd like to do and see yourself doing it. Then do it! Remember that you are strong and that you can now experience the joy of participating in life. You no longer have to be a bystander in the activities you've only watched.

- Make exercise more pleasurable by listening to good music or watching television. Get other members of your family involved, such as children, who may enjoy being active with you.

- During exercise, gently push yourself to reach your target heart rate, which is about 60 to 85 percent of your maximum heart rate. To figure out your maximum heart rate, subtract your age from 220. The remainder is your *maximum* heart rate. Do *not* attempt to reach your maximum heart rate! Use this number to find your target heart rate. To find this number, multiply your maximum heart rate by 0.6 or by 0.85. This will give you a good target range.

  If you don't know your target zone, you'll know you're in the right zone for you if you're "huffing and puffing." However, if you cannot talk or have a lot of difficulty breathing, chances are you've exceeded your target zone and need to slow it down or stop and rest.

- For maximum benefit, exercise within your target heart range for at least twenty to thirty minutes three times a week. You can break this up into two or three ten-minute intervals each day and get the same results as one twenty- or thirty-minute session. While it may be difficult for you to exercise for a full ten minutes at first, be sure to start somewhere. Begin with one minute if necessary; then build on that by gently pushing yourself.

- During exercise, as well as all throughout the day, it is essential to stay hydrated. Water should be your beverage of choice during exercise. If you feel week, dizzy, nauseated, or if your heart rate has exceeded your target zone, you are probably dehydrated. Don't wait until you feel thirsty to drink. That's too late. Instead, sip water periodically while you exercise to avoid dehydration.

- When you are engaging in resistance training, be sure to rotate your muscle groups. That is, work on a different set of muscles every other day. Take a day of rest between workouts. So, for instance, you might work on your upper body on Monday, rest on Tuesday, work on your abdominal region on Wednesday, rest on Thursday, work on your lower-body muscles on Friday, rest on Saturday, and begin the cycle again on Sunday. It's important to take your day of rest seriously. This gives your muscles a chance to repair themselves, which actually strengthens and builds the muscle!

- If you have begun strength training, you may need more than the recommended 60 to 80 grams of protein. Adequate protein intake will help you prevent loss of muscle mass and build more muscle. It will also help your body heal faster and provide it with the energy it needs. If you're not getting enough protein and you're losing muscle mass as a result, a body fat analysis should bring this to light. See the inset "Body Fat Analysis" below.

- Not all exercise has to be structured. You can increase your physical activity by taking care of "chores," such as housework, gardening, washing your car, and taking your dog for a walk. You can also participate in enjoyable physical activities. For example, run around with your children or a friend's child, chase your dog, have a game of toss, go fly a kite, punch a punching bag, play badminton, or anything else you can think of. Watch how kids play at a park to get an idea of how else you can increase your physical activities. Consider taking a weekly walk or hike with a friend. Talk while you walk and the time will fly by as your friendship deepens. The possibilities are truly endless!

Body-Fat Analysis

Some people may be delighted to have lost 100 pounds six months after surgery. However, without exercise, 60 pounds of that can be attributed to muscle loss. Muscle is essential to help ensure weight-loss maintenance for the rest of your life. The first six months are critical for maintaining the lean body mass you had before surgery. That's why it's so important to exercise regularly and maintain an adequate protein intake.

In our office, we periodically interpret our patients' weight loss by performing a body-fat analysis to make sure they are losing fat mass, not muscle mass. A body-fat analysis should be done at three-month intervals to evaluate your protein intake as well as your level of exercise to determine if it's enough for you. By monitoring a patient's body fat, we can make sure he is exchanging muscle mass for fat mass and explain the results to the patient. Hopefully, this will motivate him to continue to exercise and eat properly.

- Take up a new sport, such as tennis, the martial arts, basketball, or skiing. Don't worry if you're not good at it! Learn to laugh at your mistakes. Eventually, you're bound to getter better at it, and you'll have a good time learning.

- Enjoy your new body and the confidence you will attain as a result of your improved mobility, strength, balance, and coordination!

POSTSURGICAL MEDICAL OFFICE VISITS

For your safety and optimum results, it is in your best interest to make and keep your follow-up appointments with your surgeon. Even if you live some distance away from your surgeon's office, you need to make the effort to keep your appointments by planning ahead. This may include travel and hotel arrangements, taking time off from work, and arranging for childcare and pet care.

Although it varies, your first follow-up appointment will usually occur a week to ten days after your surgery. In some cases, it will take place around three to four weeks from the date of your surgery. In other cases, you'll be seen twice by this time. It is up to you to get precise instructions concerning when your surgeon wishes to see you after your surgery. Make your appointments early to avoid getting shut out since any surgeon's schedule can get booked up rather quickly.

At your first follow-up appointment, you'll be weighed, and your surgeon will check the site of your surgical incision(s). He may remove any sutures or staples and replace them with sterile skin closure strips such as Steri-strips. Also, he may run some blood tests. If you still have one, your G-tube may be removed at this point.

Be sure to discuss with your surgeon the need for nutritional supplements if you haven't already been started on them. Once again, tell your surgeon which medications and supplements you've been taking. (Have your updated list handy.) In fact, it's a good idea to review any medications or supplements you are currently taking at *every* appointment.

If you still have your gallbladder, your surgeon may start you on Actigall, a medication that helps prevent gallstones, since you're more at risk for developing them during your period of massive weight loss. Any number of other things may happen at your first follow-up appointment. They are all important, so be sure not to miss this appointment for any reason.

At your next appointment, you will once again be weighed in, your abdominal wounds will be checked again, and you'll undergo additional examinations. Blood may be drawn once again. Also, your surgeon will review with you how well you are eating, drinking, and exercising, and will discuss advancing your diet and exercise program.

Whenever you see your surgeon, whether it is your first visit or your tenth, tell him about any abnormal bowel movements, nausea or vomiting, pain, or other problems you are experiencing. Make a note of important instructions and information you receive from your surgeon during your visits to avoid having to call the office for clarification later on.

After your first few office visits, you'll need to make a series of appointments to see your surgeon. These are usually scheduled at three months, six months, nine months, one year, eighteen months, two years, and every year thereafter for the rest of your life. If you have problems that need special attention or are at risk for any health problems, you may need to see your surgeon more frequently.

"The rest of your life" means just that. Seeing your surgeon regularly is an essential part of your long-term health and weight loss. You've made a lifetime commitment that must be kept. Feeling good is no excuse not to keep your scheduled appointments. It is always possible that your surgeon may discover some problem that you were unaware of. This early detection may save you major problems later on.

CONCLUSION

This chapter has covered quite a bit. That's because a lot is going to be happening in those first six months following your surgery. You've come a long way, haven't you? Your body has been changing almost daily and your strength is increasing. You've found new activities to participate in and you've been getting regular exercise. You've also kept a close watch on your nutrient and fluid intake. You see your surgeon as scheduled and things are proceeding smoothly. What next? Read on to find out what happens from six months and beyond.

PART THREE

Your Future—
Thin and Healthy
for Life

CHAPTER 10

$\mathcal{S}$IX MONTHS AND BEYOND

Can you believe six months have passed since your surgery? You are probably feeling better physically—your energy is returning and your comorbidities have diminished significantly. You've most likely seen a surprising and substantial weight loss. You are still concerned about your physical body, but other concerns have begun to surface as you look toward the future. While you probably feel calmer and more centered much of the time, you may still have days when your emotions are all over the place. This is not uncommon since your body is rapidly changing and a lot of other things around you are also changing. These changes can sometimes be confusing and disorienting.

For most people who have had weight-loss surgery, losing weight was a dream that goes as far back as they can remember. *What would life be like if I were thin?* was always at the back of their minds. Over the years, you probably also had dreams and thoughts about a new, streamlined you. Now, with weight-loss surgery as a powerful tool, this new you has begun to emerge. While this is happening, don't lose sight of your dreams. They are a special part of who you are, so it's important to keep them in mind to guide you on your upcoming journey. You will work hard to make some of your dreams come true, while recognizing that other dreams you've had may not come to pass. You'll need to handle these disappointments and move on. This is your second chance, and it is difficult to see in advance what it will bring. Only one thing is certain: your life will be changing.

In this chapter, we'll explore the physical changes you'll be experiencing and will address some of your questions about what's happening to your body. (In later chapters, we'll take a look at the emotional aspects of what's to come.) Although your journey is unique to you, our aim is to provide you with a road map of sorts that will help guide you through some of the common fears and confusion people usually have while they are going through these changes. You have a right to be a little scared. You have been given a second chance. Approaching your new tomorrow with commitment, hope, support, and most of all curiosity will make it an exciting ride into an equally exciting future.

WILL I LOSE TOO MUCH WEIGHT?

Rest assured; you won't keep losing weight until you become unnaturally thin. The reason is quite simple. You will only continue to lose weight until the number of calories you take in each day equals the number of calories your body burns each day. As discussed in the previous chapter, for the first six or so months after the surgery, the average weight-loss-surgery

---

Weight-Loss Matters

As you now know, the amount of weight you are likely to lose and how quickly you lose it depends on the type of surgery you had and how your body behaves in response to the changes. People who have been fitted with inflatable bands usually lose weight the slowest and for the longest period of time. This is because most surgeons these days prefer to inflate the band slowly to produce a more gradual weight loss that can last for up to three years.

With other weight-loss procedures, the loss is usually more rapid, with a loss of about 10 to 15 pounds per month or so during the first few months, depending on various factors. The weight loss levels off in about one to two years. The leveling off tends to work by halves. For example, if you lose 45 pounds in the first three months, at the end of the next three months, you will lose about half that, or about 22 pounds. At the end of the following three months, you'll lose about 11 pounds, then 5, then 2, then 1. This, of course, is not an exact science.

If you stop losing weight prematurely, speak with your surgeon. You may need to decrease the amount of calories you're taking in and increase your physical activities. Also, your surgeon will probably want to check your stomach pouch to make sure that nothing has gone wrong. Be sure to keep in mind that weight loss occurs as a series of plateaus—you lose weight, it levels off, and then you lose some more. Don't be alarmed if you plateau. It is

patient takes in about 500 to 800 calories a day. She may burn about twice that amount or more depending upon her starting weight.

As long as your body keeps burning more calories than you eat, you will continue to lose weight. Keep in mind, however, that after a large amount of weight loss, your body will become more efficient at holding on to the calories you consume. Like most weight-loss-surgery patients, you'll probably burn about 10 to 25 percent fewer calories each day than a person who never had a weight problem. Therefore, at your reduced body size, you'll burn far fewer calories at six months and beyond than you did in the earlier months following your surgery. At the same time, you'll be able to take in an increasing number of calories each day.

When the greater number of calories you eat matches the fewer calories your body burns each day—that is, calories *in* equals calories *out*—your

---

important to continue to comply with your program and not be discouraged. If you maintain compliance, you will begin to lose again.

Weight loss also depends on how much you snack or graze between meals as well as how much exercise you get, what medications you take, the frequency of your bowel movements, the amount of fluid retention, and the time of the month in the case of women. The bottom line is, no one can predict exactly when or how much weight you'll lose at any given time.

About 15 to 20 percent of the weight-loss-surgery patients who fail to lose the expected weight are either "snackers" or "gorgers." They also tend to eat frequent, irregular meals. For instance, at about a year or two after surgery, some people develop a strong craving to snack, sometimes almost continuously, on sugary foods. Snackers have more difficulty losing weight than gorgers, since gorgers tend to vomit the large amounts of food that their small stomachs cannot handle. Both of these eating behaviors are destructive habits. If you should develop either of these problems, we urge you to seek professional help immediately.

In one to four years after the weight levels off, some people may gain back about 5 to 10 percent of their weight. The reason for this mild increase is usually due to their becoming more efficient at eating or their stomach pouch has stretched. To keep this in check, increase your level of exercise and go for nutritional counseling. Rest assured, though, long-term follow-up of people who have undergone weight-loss surgery reveals that the majority of them keep the weight off long term.

body will be in a state of "calorie balance." This is when your weight loss levels off to zero. This usually happens when the calorie intake per day averages about 1,200 to 1,300 calories for women and about 1,500 to 1,600 calories for men. With this in mind, a warning is in order: If a woman who has had weight-loss surgery takes in 1,200 or more calories a day, she will most likely gain some weight a year or so down the road. For men, weight gain can occur around the 1,500 or more calories per day mark. (Note, however, that engaging in regular exercise will help your body burn 100 or more calories each day than it normally would. Of course, the exact amount of calories you'll burn depends upon the intensity of your exercise, the number of times per week you exercise, and the length of time for each session. In any event, if you exercise regularly, you could conceivably take in a few more calories without gaining weight.)

WILL I BECOME MALNOURISHED?

The key to not becoming malnourished as a result of your surgery lies in consuming enough protein to meet your daily goals and taking good-quality vitamin and mineral supplements. Review the discussions on postsurgical nutrition throughout this book and speak with your nutritionist so you are clear on how much of the various nutrients you should consume daily.

When malnutrition does become a problem in an otherwise uncomplicated case, it usually occurs around six, nine, or twelve months or more after the surgery. This problem begins to develop when people do not regularly take their protein and other supplements or when the body does not adequately absorb these substances. The most common early sign of malnutrition is swelling (or edema) of the feet, ankles, and legs, in a manner that is abnormal for that particular individual. (By the way, edema could also be a symptom of kidney or heart problems, as well as other problems, so be sure to see a doctor about any abnormal swelling.)

A simple blood test can make the diagnosis. If serum albumin, a protein, is in the range of 2.5 grams percent or less, the swelling is likely related to malnutrition. In a case such as this, hospitalization may be needed for intravenous nutrition, also called *intravenous hyperalimentation* (IVH), which is a method of providing all the necessary nutrients directly into your body through your veins.

You'll certainly want to avoid becoming malnourished, so follow your nutritionist's recommendations very carefully and meet with her periodically. When you reach the six-month mark, you'll be eating many different types of foods. Be sure to make protein a main part of your diet. If you are still limited in the protein foods you can eat—for example, if you can't eat red meat without experiencing feedback—pay special attention to other protein sources suggested by your nutritionist.

WHERE ARE THESE SWEET CRAVINGS COMING FROM?

When your weight starts to level off or sometime later, your cravings for sweets and other high-carbohydrate foods will likely return or develop for the first time. It's not entirely clear why this occurs. If it happens to you, know that you haven't done anything wrong. It may simply be a result of your biochemistry. An amino acid supplement that is available at most health stores, 5-hydroxytryptamine, may help reduce your sugar cravings. If you wish to try it, follow the recommendations on the label. Your surgeon's office may recommend products containing artificial sweeteners, sugar-free syrups, and other foods that can help you deal with the cravings, at least to some extent.

By all means, discuss your cravings with your surgeon before taking any steps. It's important to keep her updated about what's happening to your body. Although it is not usual, your cravings may indicate a problem, such as the pouch's reconnection with the bypassed stomach. This is a very serious matter, since this reconnection enables you to eat and absorb more food than before. You could wind up regaining much of the weight you worked so hard to lose. In certain cases, the only treatment for this complication is reoperation, along with all the associated risks. Once again, your surgeon should provide you with all of the information you need to be a well-informed patient.

HOW DO I STAY ON COURSE IF PHYSICAL HUNGER RETURNS WITH A VENGEANCE?

For the first twelve to eighteen months following your surgery, you will likely feel little physical hunger. Until that time, what you may have been feeling is called *head hunger*—a combination of your body's expecting to be fed and a sense of feeling deprived, as well as the mind's grieving for what it can no longer eat. However, physically, a small amount of food will fill you up, and if you do overeat, you will experience unpleasant side effects, such as feedback and dumping syndrome. Unfortunately, this "grace period" lasts for only a short period of time.

After the first year or year and a half—or sometimes a little later—you will be able to eat more food without discomfort. And, for many, hunger returns with unexpected ferocity. If this happens to you, it is important not to panic or come to think that this is just another "yo-yo" diet and give up. Remember, this is *not* just another diet—you have worked hard to reach this place, and you will continue to comply with your program and maintain your health and weight loss. Be prepared for this phase, so that when it does occur, you can continue to lose weight and maintain your health. The following tips may help.

- Develop proper eating habits early on in the process. Once established, these habits will keep you on the straight and narrow when your cravings return or when you reach a plateau. Healthy eating habits include learning what satiety feels like—in other words, recognizing and acknowledging when you really are hungry and when you feel full. By this time, you will have learned to read your body's cues and can stop eating when your stomach sends you its "I'm-full" message. This is the ultimate in portion control. Simply don't eat when you are not hungry.

- Continue to eat three to six times a day, per your surgeon's recommendations. Continue to take small bites of food and, if possible, use smaller utensils and dishes. Chew your food fully and completely. This will help you to savor the taste and texture of what you are eating so you can enjoy your food that much more.

- Don't sample food while cooking and preparing it. Wait for mealtimes.

- Eat only at the table—not in the car, in bed, out of the refrigerator, or from the kitchen counter. Spend at least twenty to thirty minutes at the table.

- Eat your protein-rich foods first. Then, eat other foods until you begin to feel full. Remember not to drink during your meals.

- Don't finish leftovers from serving dishes or your children's plates. It's okay to throw out food, despite what you might have been told as a child. Alternatively, store leftovers in the refrigerator for another meal.

- Avoid buffets, all-you-can-eat restaurants, wine tastings, free food samples, and potluck dinners. When visiting friends for a meal, don't hesitate to remind your hostess what you can and cannot eat, or bring an approved dish with you, if necessary.

- Avoid grazing—a sure road to weight gain. Eating small amounts throughout the day can sometimes fool your stomach pouch, but it will prove disastrous. You will have fooled no one but yourself. Remember, you are in control.

- Keep vitamins and other supplements in plain view.

- Make an appointment with your nutritionist to discuss your meal plans.

- Ask support group members for help. They know how easy it is to become complacent when you approach your goal weight. They'll help you through it.

HOW DO I DEAL WITH HARMFUL PRESURGICAL EATING HABITS?

Destructive behaviors, like compulsive overeating, binge eating, and grazing will not magically stop after the surgery—although the fear of dumping syndrome and loss of appetite initially serve as deterrents. While almost everyone has used food at some point to cope with the difficulties of life, this type of behavior is different. For many of our patients, food is their drug of choice. The thin line between using food to comfort or ease negative feelings and eating disorders has to do with how much, how often, and in what ways food is used. It also has to do with the compulsive pull toward the negative behaviors as well as with a feeling of being out of control or unable to stop the behavior. You have waited a long time for this second chance. If you feel you cannot control your destructive presurgical eating patterns, seek immediate help. Start by calling your surgeon's office. They will probably recommend a therapist who can meet with you individually or in a group setting. Discuss these issues with people in your support group; some of them are probably going through the same thing. Overeaters Anonymous and similar groups are also valuable resources.

ARE MEDICAL FOLLOW-UPS REALLY NECESSARY?

After the initial follow-up appointments, some surgeons recommend follow-up visits every six months for life. Others recommend yearly visits. While this may seem to you like an unnecessary bother, these follow-ups are extremely important for making sure there are no undetected complications or problems. We can't emphasize enough how essential it is to continue seeing your surgeon—or someone with similar experience and skills—for life. During these visits, you will be weighed, your interval history will be taken, you will be examined, and you will probably undergo some blood tests.

Blood tests can tell us a lot, often well in advance of physical signs that something is wrong. Some people have, unfortunately, waited until they had an obvious problem before following up with their surgeon and had to be admitted to the hospital. To prevent unnecessary suffering and expense, we recommend that at least once a year, our patients undergo a full blood count and screening tests for salt levels in the blood, increased levels of nitrogen in the blood, or poor clearance of a muscle breakdown product called *serum creatinine.* In addition, studies of liver enzymes, calcium, phosphorus, magnesium, zinc, albumin, vitamin A, vitamin D, and vitamin B_{12} are also useful. In the case of an abnormality, further tests may be needed to study the problem further. Moreover, if a person had elevated blood fats before surgery, it's wise to keep track of the levels later on. It's not uncommon for cholesterol and trigylceride levels to be lower for a couple of years following surgery only to become elevated again in later years, especially following restrictive bariatric surgeries such as gastric banding or gastroplasty.

If there's a reason to suggest the need for it, your surgeon may take x-rays or a scope exam of your intestinal tract at any one of your follow-up appointments. You'll also be examined for problems, such as a hernia. These regular appointments also give you the opportunity to discuss any concerns you have and the opportunity to review any medication you are taking.

No matter how well you are feeling, don't miss seeing your surgeon at least once a year. This will ensure long-term weight-loss success and continued health. In addition, your surgeon and staff will be pleased to share your progress with you.

WHAT CAN BE DONE ABOUT SAGGING SKIN?

It's not uncommon for the skin to sag following massive weight loss. How much it sags is a very individual issue that depends mostly on how much elastin your skin contains. As the name suggests, elastin is a protein that helps maintain the skin's elasticity, thereby keeping it youthful looking. As we age, elastin breaks down without being replaced. How much elastin you were born with, how quickly it has broken down, how much your former size stretched out your skin, and how much weight you've lost, all add up to how much your skin will sag, if at all.

Many people are curious to know if regular exercise will help shrink back their skin. We can't say for sure how much exercise will help in this regard. Once again, this depends on many factors, including age, weight, and genetics.

Some people may decide to have cosmetic, or plastic, surgery. If you

---

Get Physical!

Now more than ever, getting regular daily exercise is extremely important. At this point, you've probably increased your intake of food, so increase your activities too! Physical activity burns extra calories, speeds up your metabolism for several hours following exercise, increases the body's sensitivity to insulin, and helps build and keep your muscle from wasting away. This helps burn even more calories and results in more weight loss or weight maintenance. It also produces positive effects in cases of diabetes, increased fat levels in the blood, high blood pressure, and depression. As you know, weight-loss surgery is only a diet aid. That goes for exercise, too. Having the surgery enabled you to lose enough weight so that you could exercise comfortably. So, get exercising, and do it for life!

---

want to go this route, wait until at least one and a half years have passed since your surgery or at least three months after your weight loss has completely leveled off, whichever comes later. With all the nutritional stress and changes your body has experienced, you'll want to avoid putting it through another surgery before adequate healing time has passed and your body has reached its new, healthier balance. We'll take a closer look at plastic surgery in Chapter 11.

WHAT WILL HAPPEN TO MY BYPASSED STOMACH?

Many people who've had weight-loss surgery are curious to know what happens to their bypassed stomach as time passes. As far as we know, from studying the stomach-lining samples we've taken from patients when the opportunity presented itself two to three years after the surgery, the bypassed stomach remains in basically the same condition it was in at the time of surgery. We have no good reason to expect that this will be any different fifteen, twenty, or thirty years in the future. However, at this time, no one can say for certain what changes, if any, the bypassed stomach will go through as time passes.

WHY AM I STILL GETTING SICK?

Nausea, vomiting, diarrhea, and abdominal pain are relatively common complications for the first six months following surgery. Although one or more of these problems may persist to some extent, they should be pretty much resolved by the time you reach the six-month mark. If you are still experiencing them frequently, it's important not to assume, or pretend, that nothing is wrong. You must see your surgeon to discuss whether or not what you are experiencing is normal and, if so, why. If it's not normal, your surgeon will need to figure out what may be causing it and whether or not you need treatment. Be sure to discuss all the treatment options available to you.

AM I AT RISK FOR SMALL BOWEL OBSTRUCTION?

About 2 percent of weight-loss surgery patients develop small bowel obstruction, also called *locked bowels*. The first signs usually include abdominal pains and nausea, followed later by vomiting and an absence of bowel movements for a day or longer. This complication can occur at any time in about 2 in 100 patients and can even occur, though rarely, a second time (in about 2 percent of the original 2 percent of patients, or 1 in 10,000). If treated promptly with surgery, recovery is likely. Any delay in treatment is dangerous, as part of the bowel may die, which can result in a life-threatening infection.

Small bowel obstruction is not limited to people who have had weight-loss surgery. Anyone who has undergone surgery on the abdomen for any reason, including an appendectomy, is at risk for small bowel obstruction.

CAN MY SURGERY BE UNDONE?

In rare instances, some people feel it is absolutely necessary to have their weight-loss surgery reversed. In some cases, they simply cannot live with the food restrictions. In other cases, they have not adequately resolved their presurgical eating disorders and continue the destructive behavior after surgery, which can have disastrous affects. This is just one reason why people considering weight-loss surgery, particularly those with eating disorders, should see a therapist before making the decision to have weight-loss surgery.

The ability to reverse the procedure depends on the type of surgery you've had. For example, removing a gastric band involves a relatively straightforward procedure. On the other hand, a gastric bypass is undone by reattaching the stomach and intestines, and involves considerably more surgery. In all instances, it is wise to wait at least until the initial inflammation from the surgery has settled down. This makes the reversal surgery less difficult and quicker to accomplish.

Reattachment will cause some additional internal scarring, and the stomach will not look exactly like it did before surgery. However, most people who go through the reversal process will not notice any difference other than their renewed ability to eat the way the did before the surgery.

In surgeries where part of the stomach was removed, nothing can be done to replace it. However, the remaining portion of the stomach can enlarge and usually functions much like the original, complete one.

If you have your weight-loss procedure reversed, all the benefits, such as reduced appetite, will also be undone. With the ability to eat about as much as you did before surgery, you have a good chance of gaining back all your lost weight. In some cases, you may even gain more weight than you lost.

We've found that, in many instances, surgical reversal can be avoided by getting to the heart of, and correcting, the problem that prompted the individual's desire to have the surgery reversed. If the problem has an emotional origin, the intervention of a knowledgeable mental-health therapist can sometimes prove invaluable. If the problem is physical—such as an internal hernia causing sever abdominal pain, nausea, and vomiting—it can usually be fixed with further medical intervention. In either case, in our experience, once the underlying problem is dealt with, most people are willing to accept and live with their altered anatomy. After all, who wants to have two surgeries and no benefit to show for all that pain and expense?

CONCLUSION

This chapter has probably alleviated some of your concerns and clarified others. Surely, there will be even more on your mind as your body continues to go through the transformation process. This chapter dealt with mostly physical issues, as had many of the previous chapters. It's pretty clear what's going on physically—to figure it out, all you have to do is take stock of how your body feels and look in the mirror. What's going on emotionally may be another story. Turn to the next chapter to get a close-up look at the most important part of this journey—you.

CHAPTER 11

$\mathcal{Y}$OUR MOST IMPORTANT RELATIONSHIP

The One You Have With Yourself

As you move through the weeks and months following your surgery, the enormity of your new life will hit you with full force. You will be going through so many changes that you'll sometimes feel like a stranger even to yourself. As you change on the outside, you'll be changing on the inside, too. To make the most of these changes, you'll need to redefine the relationship you have with yourself and get to know who you are all over again. To achieve long-term success, it's important to realize and understand that inner adjustments will be necessary. This chapter will help you make these adjustments so that your inner you can catch up with the outer you.

This new life will have exciting possibilities, but also challenging and essential limits. Some of these limits will be difficult. Much will be different. There will be times when you will want to test these limits. Be careful. You, and only you, are responsible for your long-term success. You can do it! Remember this is not just another diet. This is forever, and, for long-term success, compliance is essential. So, let's start there.

THE KEY TO LONG-TERM COMPLIANCE

You, more than anyone else, know that "getting with the program" doesn't mean a new food plan or exercise program. You have already tried dozens of new food plans. In fact, if you are like many of our patients, you may already be an expert on diets, calories, and the happenings at local gyms. You have already found that, while these programs helped you to lose weight, you'd only gain it back with perhaps additional pounds to show for it. Exercise programs were rarely long term, partly because of the restrictions placed on you by your weight and, often, by your pain. Long-term compliance—and certainly "forever compliance"—was just not possible for you before the surgery.

So, what is the key to long-term compliance? Let's start with the concept we call the *food mind*—the part of the mind that deals with and focuses on the importance of eating and food in every aspect of one's life. Only in understanding this important food mind can you begin to modify your behavior and your eating habits.

While food issues and eating habits are highly individual, they may not be as unique as you think. The sections to follow will help you examine, at least in part, what your relationship with food has meant to you—in other words, it will give you a look into your food mind. We'll briefly examine what is likely to happen as this relationship changes and evolves. We'll explore with you creative ways of handling these changes to maximize long-term weight-loss success and health.

FOOD—AM I GIVING UP MY BEST FRIEND?

Before surgery, one of your biggest concerns may have been what you'll be able to eat—or won't be able to eat—for the rest of your life. Food limitations are often a key concern for many people. Along with that concern often comes the important question: "When it comes to food, will I be giving up my best friend?" Our answer to this question is always an emphatic "No!" You don't have to give up food and eating at all. Rather, the nature of your relationship with food will be undergoing dramatic, beneficial changes. In the past, the issues you had with food may have seemed difficult, confusing, and shameful. Maybe you had never spoken about these issues and, as a result, felt totally alone. But this time around, you are *not* alone. You have a support system, which includes this book.

Our patient Tom talks about his relationship with food: "I was afraid that I would be without the one thing that defined my life: cooking. I loved to be in the kitchen, creating tasty dishes for my family and friends. Food was my one and only creative accomplishment; it was my hobby. Despite my considerable success with work and family, food distinguished me the most. It was a great leap of faith for me to agree to the surgery, but my weight was killing me." After his significant weight loss, Tom says, "More than 200 pounds of my relationship with food is gone. I now have a mature, non-dependent relationship with food. I still love to be around food, to be in the kitchen creating meals. Yes, cooking is still my creative outlet. I cook, I eat well, and I maintain compliance with my plan. I enjoy food—but better than that, I enjoy life!"

Like Tom, you too will find that you can still cook and enjoy food. The quantities and varieties will be different, but the opportunity for enjoyment will still be available to you. As we move on, keep Tom's poignant words in mind: *I enjoy food—but better than that, I enjoy life!*

FOOD MASKS FEELINGS—UNCOVER THEM!

Eating food masks feelings. Pain, fear, jealously, competition, sadness, loneliness, and abandonment are all common emotional triggers for overeating. Anger is also a powerful trigger: "I had plenty to be angry about," Tina told us. "I was harassed, teased, or ignored for as long as I can remember because of my weight. As a kid, I couldn't understand why people were so cruel to me. I couldn't believe how much it hurt. I kept it all in, smiled, and ate. Food masked my hurt feelings, and, for a little while, it made me feel better. Food—not those cruel people—was my friend." For Lisa, thinking about food helped her deal with frustration and insecurity at the office. She recalls, "Whenever I was having a particularly long and difficult day at work, I'd find myself thinking about what I'd do in the evening. The choice was always the same: Chinese or Italian."

No matter what feelings you were experiencing in the past, you may have found that specific combinations of high-carbohydrate, high-fat, and sugar-rich foods seemed to make the feelings disappear as if by magic, leaving a sense of psychological calm and relief from those powerful emotions. For a brief while, you may have even imagined that gorging or bingeing on food made you happy. As you learned, that particular kind of happiness was, unfortunately, fleeting. By the next day, you probably felt even worse—perhaps weak and out of control, and maybe like you'd failed again. Even more important, by masking all of these difficult feelings, you weren't able to resolve or understand them. The feelings didn't magically disappear. They were temporarily shelved only to return at a later time, resulting in renewed internal chaos, disruptions in work and relationships, and increased episodes of bingeing or gorging.

Now that your surgery is over, those feelings have a chance to be resolved. It's time to take those feelings off the shelf permanently! How can you do this? Read on.

Let Your Feelings Come

After surgery, many of our patients encounter a confusing array of intense feelings—feelings concerning not only their bodies and the surgery, but also *everything* around them. Some of the feelings that are now bubbling to the surface were buried long ago, successfully covered by layers of food. This time around, the feelings cannot be muted or masked by the intake of large amounts of food. It is likely that this will be a difficult time for you. It is critical that you learn how to handle these feelings and do not retreat from the feelings that emerge. They will give you important information about yourself, your past journeys, and your future path.

Find a quiet, peaceful place where you can spend a little time each day by yourself. Get comfortable and clear your mind of your daily routine happenings. Let the feelings come. If you can't attach words to what is going on inside you or identify the feelings at first, don't be surprised. Understanding what you're feeling may take a while. Since you are intentionally letting your feelings come to you, you may find it easier to deal with whatever you experience without the fear you may have felt in the past.

A word of caution about anger is in order here: You may be surprised by the amount of anger that emerges from inside you. Feelings of anger are not unusual in postsurgical patients, since many of them had a lot to be angry about in the past. At this point, it is important to understand the anger and to know that you aren't going crazy. Rather, you may be reexperiencing pain from the past. Learn to channel the anger in the right direction; this may involve avoiding vulnerable people around you who might become targets. If your anger feels too intense or out of control, help from a mental-health specialist, even short term, can help you understand the anger and come to a resolution.

Approach all of your feelings with curiosity. This will give you valuable clues not only about where you've come from but also about where you're going. Be gentle with yourself as the feelings emerge. Don't judge or evaluate them. Remember, there is little black and white in the world. Look for the shades of gray. All of this is a part of the new and improved you.

Talk About Your Feelings With Others

If your feelings become too intense, don't hesitate to ask for help. Speak to a family member or friend. You may already know exactly who you can turn to. In some cases, you may have distanced yourself from anyone who might help. If this is the case, you might consider reconnecting with an old friend or relative. You may be surprised by how understanding and helpful this person can be as you relate what you've been experiencing. If not, try again with someone else.

Also, members of your support group can serve as invaluable resources during this difficult period. Many of them have felt the way you are feeling. They can help you understand what you are experiencing and share with you how they have coped by using certain non-food-related ways of dealing with their feelings. This process of reaching out and sharing feelings not only provides on-the-spot relief, but also helps form a bridge to new and healthier friendships, while previously intense thoughts of food increasingly fade.

Write or Draw About Your Feelings in a Journal

You may find it useful to keep a journal in which you can record your feelings and thoughts. While you're recovering from your surgery, you might want to write in it every day. Later, you may wish to write every few days, if not every day. This journal is for your eyes only so don't worry yourself about things like style or grammar or who might see it. If you don't feel like writing, draw instead. If you don't want to draw, just splash some colors across the page.

Your "feelings diary" will serve three purposes. First, it will help you put words or images or colors to what may, at times, seem like a tangled web of emotions. Second, putting things on paper often creates a sense of increased calm and control, which makes it easier to take action. And third, in the years ahead, your journal will serve as a reminder of your early post-surgical days, helping guide you in the future when you find it difficult to comply with your plan or feel that you are losing direction.

Get Professional Help to Identify Your Feelings

Counseling sessions provide a time and place for you to learn about the most important subject in the world—you! When changes are taking place, it's often helpful to speak with a mental-health professional about what is occurring and how it is affecting you. A knowledgeable therapist, one with a background in weight-loss surgery, can provide invaluable assistance in helping you sort out what's going on inside you and identify what you're feeling. This person can help you understand and resolve past issues that may be clouding your way.

CREATING CALM AND REMOVING STRESSORS WITHOUT FOOD

For many, the intake of food relieves stress and creates inner calm. "For a long time I used food—my best friend—as a form of self-medication," said Erica. "When the world became too stressful, I carved out quiet times for myself by bingeing, to shut off my own thinking. High-calorie, high-fat foods gave me pleasure, and I soon found that eating them was almost automatic and trance-like. I began to withdraw more and more into food, shutting off the world around me."

The reality is, we all live in a highly stressful world—at home, at work, and in our communities. But, for the obese, these everyday stresses are magnified. For example, on the job, a morbidly obese person may have to work twice as hard to prove himself in an effort to dispel the appalling misconception that obese people are lazy or just "not as good" as the next person. Moreover, excess weight may cause difficult issues in relationships with family members and friends. Some obese people report having to try harder at relationships by always being kind, giving, and nice, essentially a "pushover," even in the face of indifference, mistreatment, or abuse. Furthermore, physical stresses are always present as the comorbidities of obesity increase. We certainly don't have to tell anyone who is morbidly obese about the stress of living in constant pain or with sleep apnea, which leaves one constantly exhausted and unable to function because of fatigue. The stress-reducing benefits of exercise and other activities get more and more out of reach as your extra weight interferes with your ability to do them. Stress mounts. Isolation increases. Food is there to console and calm. It's a vicious cycle.

"Food comforted me," Tina told us. "I used it to ease my feelings of inferiority and self-doubt. I used it to bury my feelings of shame and self-loathing, which resulted mostly from years of physical and sexual abuse. I began to see eating food as an addiction, much like drinking alcohol or doing drugs. When I stopped turning to alcohol for comfort in my early twenties, my food addiction took an even greater hold. I guess I just switched addictions."

Like Erica, Tina used food to escape from stress, however temporary. In Tina's case, though, the stakes were much higher. Her food issues were very much rooted in the past, as they are for many people. Unfortunately, many of our obese patients have suffered sexual and emotional abuse in their earlier years; for some, this abuse began at a very young age. In these cases, food provided them with much-needed comfort. Our patients are often surprised and relieved to learn that compulsive eating in childhood actually helped them, as children, cope with the abuse they were subjected to and prevented more serious long-term psychological problems from developing. However, postsurgically, it's essential that people with these food issues, in particular, realize (with professional help, as necessary) that they are indeed safe and that their trance-like overeating mechanism is no longer needed. In some cases, when food is no longer available to numb these painful past experiences, the feelings and memories that emerge postsurgically can be quite overwhelming. In Tina's case, psychotherapy helped her deal with her serious childhood issues and, eventually, resolve them. As a result, she was able to form a positive long-term relationship.

The feelings of calm and relief that come from eating certain foods are not imagined. We are only now beginning to get a clear picture of the changes in brain chemistry that occur when combinations of high-carbohydrate, high-fat, and sugar-rich foods are eaten. Specific food combinations can raise the levels of the calming brain chemicals tryptophan and serotonin, which can create a very real sense of calm. So, what happens when you can no longer use food to quiet your painful emotions? Read on to find out how to produce calm and reduce stress in your life without turning to food.

Reevaluate Your Stressors

Here are a few examples of what we hear from many of our "stressed-out" patients: *My kids are driving me crazy. My husband shouts all the time. Work is so demanding. I don't make enough money. I never have enough time. So many people depend on me.* Chances are you have these or similar stressors in your life.

When you resume your everyday tasks, some of the stressors you may have been able to avoid during your recovery return. This will likely trigger a desire to overeat to make them easier for you to deal with, but you know that this is no longer possible. Instead, spend some time thinking about the things that you find most stressful. Make a list in your journal, with the most serious stressors at the top of the list. Review the list and figure out which of them you can change.

In response to this suggestion, many of our patients claim that changing their lives is just not possible. We remind them that by undergoing the surgery, they have already begun to change their lives. So, the question is, what *else* can and must be changed to bring more peace into your life? Be honest with yourself when reviewing your list. Keep in mind that you, and you alone, are in control. Change *is* possible even if you find it difficult at times.

Ask yourself the following questions: Where and how can I begin to make the necessary change? Do I need help making these changes? Who can help me? Friends, family members, support group members, a therapist, my boss, my kids, a teacher, a religious person—these are just a few among the many possible people you can turn to for advice and support.

Protect Yourself

You may be very good at protecting the people you care for but not so good at protecting yourself. What does it mean to protect yourself? This includes a number of things: 1) Protecting your time by learning to say "no" when necessary to other people's requests and demands; 2) Protecting your physical and emotional space by letting others know when they have crossed your boundaries; and 3) Protecting yourself by avoiding people who are toxic and hurtful.

In most cases, you can choose who you spend your time with and what you spend your time on. Sometimes, however, social obligations such as family events where you may see people who can be negative or hurtful cannot be avoided without creating even more stress. In this case, perhaps another family member can run interference on your behalf. If you work with people who are very negative, and gentle confrontation doesn't ease the situation, perhaps you can turn to your boss or the human resources department for help.

Revisit or Renew Spiritual Ties

On the most basic level, spirituality is unique for each of us, isn't it? For some, spirituality lies in one's religion or in the belief that something or someone greater than one's self helps people make sense out of our challenging world. A firm belief in God is, to many of us, a stabilizing and unifying force in our lives. Spirituality can also be found in the beauty of nature and in the world around us. Think for a few minutes about your own unique spirituality.

If you've lost touch with your spirituality, try to become more involved in those things that will reawaken it for you. If you've never been in touch with your spiritual side, consider seeking out what spirituality might mean for you. If you're already committed to a spiritual path, think about deepening that bond. Renewing or strengthening religious beliefs or spirituality can bring you solace, peace, and balance in an otherwise turbulent world.

Pamper Yourself

Pampering yourself is a wonderful stress-reliever. Getting a massage, a facial, or a manicure or pedicure can be very relaxing after a stress-filled day or week. Also, a simple soak in a warm tub can provide instant relief when more luxurious stress-relievers are not an option. Shopping for a new outfit, listening to a symphony or music you find soothing, or going to a performance are other ways you can pamper yourself. The possibilities are virtually endless. Think about something nice that you can do for yourself, and do it. You deserve it!

Be More Creative with Your Downtime

Oftentimes, after a stress-filled day or event, a long nap on the couch may seem like the most pleasant thing you could possibly do with your time. Of course, an occasional nap is fine, but try to be more creative with your downtime. For example, engage in some light exercise. Not only is exercise the key to long-term weight maintenance, it's also a great stress-reliever. Many of our patients who take this advice to get up and out rather than give in to the urge to sleep are amazed to discover that they feel less tired and less stressed after something as simple as walk around the block. With that said, be sure to listen to your body. If you are very tired, go ahead and sleep, just don't sleep excessively. If you do find yourself sleeping more than you should, call your surgeon's office for help. Sleeping all the time is a sign of depression or perhaps another significant problem that needs your surgeon's attention.

Elevate Your Other Senses

For a long time, you've relied on your sense of taste for pleasure. Of course you can still enjoy the taste of your food in smaller quantities, but now you can begin to rely more on your other senses—sight, hearing, smell, and touch—for pleasure, too. To elevate your sense of touch, consider massage or other form of bodywork; become more aware of the tender touch of a loved one. To enhance your sense of smell, try new lotions, perfumes, essential oils, incense, and bath oils. Go to a flower shop and sniff the different flowers. You can elevate your sense of sight this way too by taking in the colorful array of the petals and leaves. Consider adding new colors to your living space—and to your clothes. Slimming black clothes are no longer your only option. Be a peacock; you'll look great! Listen for new sounds or new music to increasingly develop your sense of hearing. A walk through nature can easily fill all your senses. Experiment with new things that stimulate your whole body and make it come alive! Feel your new body and the wonder of the world around you.

BODY IMAGE AND SELF-IMAGE—NEW CHALLENGES

Like many people who choose weight-loss surgery, the question "What would life be like if I were thinner?" may have always been in the back of your mind. Maybe you had fantasies about being thin and active but never thought they'd actually come true. Weight-loss surgery has given you the chance to make those fantasies a reality. A new, more streamlined you is emerging. Along with the substantial changes you're going through, your self-image and body image will be challenged, and that's to be expected. For example, Margie is an outgoing and successful businesswoman. Two years after her surgery, she's lost 120 pounds and usually seems like she's on top of the world. However, one day when she came to our office for her scheduled appointment, her usual sense of control was missing. She sat down and began to cry. "This morning, I looked in the mirror and a different face looked back. Who is she? I feel like I don't even know who I am anymore or where my life is going. So much has changed. Life is great, but I'm scared." We helped Margie begin to deal with her concerns, just as the sections to follow can help you deal with the puzzling question "Who am I now?"

Discovering Your New Identity

Food may have defined almost every aspect of your life for as long as you can remember. It may have played a part in the people you chose as friends, in your activities, in your involvement in the community, in your employment opportunities, and even in your ability to have and raise children and to marry. Food was an important part of your past identity. But now, both your weight and your relationship with food have radically changed. So, like Margie, you may very well be asking, "Who am I now?"

To begin to figure this out, it's a good idea to go to a quiet place and write in your journal. Start with a list of five positive words that describe you. Don't think about it. Just begin to write. Next, list three roles that describe you—for example, daughter, wife, mother, son, husband, father, volunteer, teacher, student, artist, and so on. Then, list five things you like to do that don't involve food. Finally, list five things that make you special and unique. If you can't think of five things, write whatever comes to mind. (You can ask a close friend or family member to help you come up with some at a later time.) Now, spend some time looking at the list. Copy it and carry it around with you in your wallet or purse and look at it every day. Food does not define you. This list does! Add to your list as you discover new things about yourself or as you listen to the feedback of others. Watch the list grow.

Keep in mind that being obese often involves putting dreams on hold. As you begin to redefine who you are, rekindle those old dreams or dream

How Funny Is That?!

Some overweight people find comfort in their identity as the jokester in their social group. You may have developed a good sense of humor at an early age to help you cope socially, even when life around you wasn't really very funny. Sometimes, you may have even poked fun at yourself as your way of coping with your size and its problems. Now is the time to turn things around. The ability to make people laugh, without being hurtful to yourself or others, is a great trait. You can take advantage of this gift by using it on yourself—that is, make yourself laugh by noticing the light-hearted humor in the world around you and inside you. As life around you changes, develop your sense of humor so that you can see the absurd and take pleasure in it. Focus on the silly! See funny movies and read cartoons. Get together with friends for a night of silliness. It's never too late to be the carefree kid you missed being. With your new energy, you'll have plenty of time to laugh, laugh, laugh. There's so much out there to enjoy!

anew. Are there things you've always wanted to do or try? People you'd like to meet or places you'd like to visit? Make your dreams a reality. Fulfilling your dreams, or at least some of them, also helps define you—adventurer, go-getter, risk-taker, seeker, tennis player, martial artist, the possibilities go on and on. So go ahead and add to your list as you discover new important things about yourself!

Body Image—It May Not Be What's in the Mirror

Everything around you may seem like it's in a continuing state of change. Your body, your meals, your relationships, your work situation, and even the very way you perceive the world may be changing. In the midst of all of this, one thing that is not changing may be your body image. In the simplest sense, the term *body image* is frequently used to describe how we feel about and see our bodies. However, the concept of body image is actually much more complex.

Adrienne Ressler, MA, CSW, National Training Director at the Renfrew Center, an acclaimed eating disorders treatment center, defines *body image* in her lectures as having three components: 1) the way you *look* at yourself in your mind's eye, 2) the way you believe others perceive you, and 3) most important, the way you actually *feel* living in your body. This definition is particularly important because it stresses the fact that your body image is, to a large degree, completely subjective—that is, it depends upon your unique perceptions and feelings about yourself. At times, this may be far different from the objective reality—how you *really* look and how others *really* see you.

"I'm still having a somewhat difficult time with my body image," Tina said. "When I look at myself in the mirror, I still see the very large me just the same as before my surgery. The scale says I'm dropping pounds and my clothes are practically falling off, so logic takes over, and my brain acknowledges that I'm losing weight. Still, it's hard for me to actually *see* it. When I found out that a new friend of mine weighs only fifteen pound less than I do, I was shocked. I thought of her as being a fairly healthy weight, but hadn't thought of myself that way. I accidentally caught our side-by-side reflection in a mirror, and broke down in tears to see that we were about the same size."

You may be like Tina. Although your weight is changing, you still feel and see your old fat when you think about your body. In clothing shops, you may find yourself heading toward the larger sizes. You sidestep mirrors and other reflective surfaces to avoid seeing yourself. These may be old habits. When you do look in the mirror and *really* see yourself, you may be startled by the body and face staring back at you.

"Even five years after my surgery, I'm still not used to how I look," David said. "I can't pass a mirror or a window without doing a double take."

Adrienne Ressler explains this phenomenon this way: You have lost weight so quickly your brain and senses just haven't had time to catch up. If you recognize yourself in Tina's and David's stories, you're probably experiencing much the same body-image distortion as they are. Body-image distortion is a very common occurrence in weight-loss-surgery patients. Although common, it can have serious consequences if left unchecked and unexamined.

In the case of many of our morbidly obese patients, their weight, their feelings about their weight, and their perceptions of their bodies formed the essence of who they were. Body image was confused with their self-esteem and self-concept, and became their complete identity—their physical bodies became them. For many, the prevalent message they were giving themselves was "I am what I weigh." Others had an even more destructive message: "I look gross; I am gross!"

Why is it so hard to change these negative images even after massive weight loss and positive feedback from others? It may not seem to make any sense at all. But it actually makes a lot of sense. On the most basic level, these destructive, hurtful, and untrue feelings about one's body and, in some cases, one's whole sense of self are difficult to change because they have been around for so long—sometimes since infancy. The following section takes a look how one's body image develops.

The Development of Body Image

Let's begin with a brief look at the first component of body image—the way you see yourself in your mind's eye. According to Ressler, body-image distortions can begin in infancy when we first begin to have a sense of our bodies through the sense of touch. The sense of touch is a paramount influence in the establishment of bonding and connecting to the external world. Invasive touch can lead to a sense of feeling "wide open," where there is no delineation between one's self and caretaker. As a result, the developing child does not know how to set limits or see himself as separate from others. This can lead to a person who wants to take in everything (such as food) and doesn't know where to draw the line. On the other hand, not enough touch can leave an infant without a sense of connection, never feeling full and always longing for more. This person wants to be cared for and loved, and so he turns to things that will give him that feeling of fullness (such as food). Most important, in both cases, the caretaker is not responding to the child's signals, and as a result, the child never learns to trust, or be in touch with, his body's signals and sensations. The result of these experiences may lead to an adolescent and adult with distorted internal body cues.

Throughout life, a person with distorted internal body cues will search outside himself for answers. This outward-seeking behavior leads to problems with the second component of body image—that is, how others perceive you or how you *think* others perceive you. From the time an infant is born, he receives verbal and non-verbal messages from the people around him about body shape, size, and appearance. Some of our patients recall family members repetitively saying what a big baby they were and how cute it was to watch them wobble around on their fat little legs or how much they liked to pinch their chubby cheeks. Others remember being called nicknames like butterball, tubby, and a wide variety of probably well-meaning but destructive identifying labels. Certainly, these labels don't cause one to become obese, but in an obese person, such labels can be very hurtful and tend to stick around. *What is your earliest memory of what you were called as a child? What messages might you have received about your body and your emerging sense of self?*

As a child grows, the verbal and non-verbal messages they receive about their bodies take on more and more significance. We've observed that children as young as age four or five are acutely conscious of body size. In many cases, as early as kindergarten, friendships and popularity are often based on appearance and weight.

Chances are you've been cutting yourself off from your body to avoid physical and emotional pain for quite some time. In effect, you might have been living from the neck up as many of our patients do. With no internal signals you could count on or understand, you learned to depend on messages you received from others, which were often distorted.

The third component of body image lies in how comfortable a person is in his own body. This is a particularly complex issue for the morbidly obese. How is it possible to be comfortable in a body that, for as long as you can remember, you've been at war with and maybe have even come to hate? How can you be comfortable in a body that does not fit into a chair in a restaurant, movie theater, or airplane? Even more important, how is it possible to be comfortable in a body with physical limitations and comorbidities, a body that frequently causes not only emotional but also physical pain?

As you transform into a healthier person, you'll eventually become more comfortable in your body. Some of your old feelings about your body will diminish with time, usually within a few years at least. Having some idea of how you developed your body-image distortion can help you understand some of the confusion. In addition, you can help to resolve old feelings and reinvent your body image by partaking in some of the creative exercises suggested in the following section.

Creating Your New Body Image

Things are about to change! Let's begin with how you see yourself in your mind's eye. How long has it been since you looked at yourself in a full-length mirror? Go ahead and take a good long look. This will help you get in touch with your feelings about your body. At first, do this with clothing on. In fact, you may want to wear a special outfit or arrange your hair just so. When you feel more comfortable at some later time, you can perform this exercise without clothing.

Scan your body from head to toe. What do you see? Listen closely for the messages you are giving yourself about your body. Think about the words you are using to describe your body. Are they positive or negative? Do any of them come from the past and simply need to be deleted from the list of words you use to describe yourself? Although you may be pleased about your weight loss, you may be surprised that many of the messages you are giving yourself are negative. You may have become accustomed to reinforcing your negative body image by almost unconsciously calling yourself names, by comparing yourself to unreal media images or body ideals. Stop giving yourself these damaging messages! Make a conscious effort to replace these negative messages with positive ones. Focus on the aspects of your body that you feel good about and reinforce those messages. For example, "I have beautiful eyes." "My skin is clear and smooth." "My arms and legs are strong." You can also change the negative messages to positive ones. For example, change "my thighs are so fat" to something like "my thighs are so strong they help me walk longer and longer distances each day." Now is the time to change your internal messages. You can do it!

Write these positive messages in your journal. Write some of them on poster board and hang them where you will see them every day. Become aware throughout the day when negative messages about your body pop into your head (you may be surprised at how often they appear). When they come, squash them and replace them with positive messages. You may want to jot down the negative messages as you become aware of them so that you can edit them in black and white into positive statements. Repeat the positive messages to yourself every day whenever you think about it.

Don't stop focusing on the positive aspects of your body. Don't rush by mirrors and reflective windows. Instead, stop to look at yourself fully and completely. This is the new you! You are learning to love your body. The sooner you learn to give yourself positive messages, the sooner you can stop relying on others for your image of your own body and, indeed, of yourself. Remember, you have worked so hard to get to this place.

Spend some time every day looking in the mirror. Revel in all of your new positive messages. This is such a simple exercise, but it's very important. You are getting to know your healthier and more beautiful body—all of it! During the "getting to know you" period, avoid compartmentalizing. In other words, when you find yourself focusing negatively on one body part, remind yourself that you are a whole person. No part of you should be singled out as good or bad. "The key is not to love every part," says Ressler, "but to accept them and realize they are all a part of you. Your thighs may not be perfect but they do the job of carrying you around."

Another simple way to help you develop a more rapid sense of your new body size is to simply run your hands over the contours of your chest, abdomen, and thighs ten times both morning and night. Pause for a moment and feel how far apart your hands are now. For another creative exercise that you and your support group can do to help improve your concept of body image, see the inset "Positive Self-Talk in a Group Setting" below.

Now, let's get in touch with how others perceive you or how you *think*

Positive Self-Talk in a Group Setting

Here's a creative exercise, described by Adrienne Ressler at a meeting of the International Association of Eating Disorder Professionals (IAEDP) Foundation, that you and your support group may want to consider trying at one of your meetings to help improve everyone's concept of body image.

Imagine that you're at a party or gathering not related to your weight issues. Bring to mind some of the negative feelings you've had, or still have, about your body. Choose a sentence to describe those feelings, beginning with the statement "I am . . ." Then, add an ending that gets your negative feelings across such as "gross," "fat," "boring," or "out of control."

Now, go around the room and shake hands with the other people. As you do, look them in the eye and voice your negative statement. Listen closely to their negative statement. Notice how these messages make you feel. You might think these messages sound absurd when voiced, but this is what you have been doing inside your head for years!

Next, choose a positive message about yourself, one that you really believe. Once again, complete the statement "I am . . ." If you have trouble coming up with something, ask the other group members for help. They'll probably have many positive messages for you.

Now, as you go around the room shaking hands, state the positive message about yourself. Say it several times during the handshake. For instance, "I am very healthy," "I am strong," "I am elegant," or "I am more powerful each day." Notice how these new messages make you feel.

When everyone has done this, gather together as a group to discuss the different feelings that surfaced depending on the message you gave and received. You may be surprised that such a simple technique can be so powerful. It reinforces a positive self-image and body image and also helps your brain and senses catch up with the actual changes that have taken place in your body.

others perceive you to remedy this aspect of body-image distortion. You might need to shift lenses here. Instead of assuming others are thinking negative things about you, listen for positive comments from those around you. Embrace these comments and take pride in them. The more weight you lose, the more frequently people may pay you compliments. Try not to be overly sensitive or misperceive what they say, since you may not be accustomed to others talking about your body in a positive way. For example, Lydia, who'd lost a great deal of weight, thought her coworker was making disparaging remarks when she commented to another worker about Lydia's weight. In reality, her coworker was happy for Lydia and had been telling other workers how proud she was of Lydia's weight-loss success.

It's completely natural for people to notice your substantial weight loss, and some will comment on what they are seeing. Not everyone is tactful. Others will ask questions out of mere curiosity. You can choose to answer the questions or just thank them for their interest. In any case, know that they are usually pleased that you've had such success. By listening for positive messages, you will be changing your concept of how others perceive you. These messages will help cancel out the old messages.

As you walk down the street, practice holding your head high (reach for the stars!). When you were obese, you may have avoided eye contact with others. But now, try to make eye contact with the people you pass. Smile at them. You may be surprised at how much of a difference that makes and how often they smile back. This is your new healthy body—wear it proudly!

How you feel in your body will be changing as your weight drops and you become more active. You'll feel healthier, stronger, and, in many cases, pain-free. The freedom from pain will be a wonderful change for some of you. This will help repair your body image quite a bit. You'll naturally feel better about living in your body, but you'll need to give yourself time to adjust to the changes. You can help your brain adjust to your body changes by becoming grounded—that is, becoming completely aware of your body and its connection to the earth. See the inset "Becoming Grounded" on page 214.

IS PLASTIC SURGERY A POSSIBLE NEXT STEP?

If you are considering plastic surgery, the first question to ask yourself is "why?" For some people, the reason is a cosmetic one. Although the primary reason for weight-loss surgery is medical, most people look forward to having a more attractive body. Plastic surgery can dramatically improve the way you look. However, for many of our patients, the reason for seeking plastic surgery is not just cosmetic.

In *Update: Surgery for the Morbidly Obese Patient* (FD-Communications, 2000), contributors Drs. Cowan, Wallace, Marx, and Hiler write: "Increasing numbers of morbidly obese patients are losing massive amounts of excess weight, due to improved long term and short term surgical results. While this permits them to reap many of the medical physical, social, psychological and economic benefits of bariatric surgery, they are often left with

Becoming Grounded

When you are completely aware of your body and its connection to the earth, it's called *being grounded*. Being aware of your body this way can help your body image catch up with the physical changes that are taking place. There are many ways to become more grounded. For example, participating in activities such as martial-arts training, yoga, and tai chi can make you much more aware of your body and how it feels to be inside it. The long-term benefits of these activities include a better sense of balance, coordination, strength, and confidence. Simple stretching exercises that you can do at home and even soaking in a bathtub with scented oils will help you tune into your body. Another simple way to become more grounded is to do the following exercise:

Stand with your legs slightly apart (about shoulder-width). Plant yourself by firmly pressing your feet into the ground with even pressure. Relax your arms and legs; don't lock your knees. Find a point or object straight ahead and gaze through it, as if an endless horizontal plane lay before you. Now, imagine that you are sending energy very slowly from the top of your head down through your body. When the energy arrives at your feet, imagine that they are like the roots of a tree deeply embedded in the ground. Embrace this feeling for a few minutes without moving—feel the energy flowing throughout your body from head to toe, and be completely aware of your connection to the earth. After a few moments, gently shake out your body and relax. You will be fully and completely in your new and healthy body.

The more you partake in exercises aimed at grounding yourself and the more familiar the feeling of being in your body becomes, the sooner your body image will catch up with all the wonderful changes that are taking place on the outside.

extremely redundant masses of skin, fat and other bodily distortions in various anatomic locations." What exactly does that mean for you? In the simplest terms, you will be losing a significant amount of weight in a relatively short time following your surgery. Some of your remaining skin will probably have some folds and not smoothly cover your new shape as well as you might like. The result may be loose, hanging skin over some parts of your body. Excessive fat may remain in other areas.

The most troublesome places are usually the abdomen, breasts, thighs, upper arms, and face. For some of our patients, this is not a significant issue; others, however, seek additional surgical correction in the form of plastic surgery. In their cases, their excess skin, fat, and tissue have gotten in the way of many daily areas of functioning. Hygiene has become an issue, creating problems of cleanliness and possible skin disease in the extra skin folds. Bacterial and fungal growth often creates unpleasant body odors despite attempts at care. Excess tissue, particularly in the abdominal area, can cause difficulty walking. Large and heavy breasts can cause neck and back pain, rubbing and chafing of the skin under the breasts, deep indentations in the skin from bra straps, difficulty exercising, and difficulty finding clothes. Loose folds of skin can embarrass some people, particularly in areas of the body that tend to be exposed to view like the upper arms and neck. Other people find themselves self-conscious in sexual situations when their outer clothing is removed. This may be particularly difficult for people who have just begun to date. All of the above are very real reasons to seek a plastic-surgery consultation. So, what's the next step?

When and How to Proceed

It is probably important to wait until your weight is stabilized before considering plastic surgery. This usually happens one year to eighteen months after surgery. Many plastic surgeons will refuse to operate if they do not feel you can maintain a weight that you are satisfied with. Ask your weight-loss surgeon for the name of a plastic surgeon who has worked with many people who have had weight-loss surgery, so that there will be expertise and respect available for your unique issues. For example, in a tummy tuck, these issues can include the possibility of finding a hernia that has gone undetected. Another important factor is that you may have a great deal more lax skin than the average person who gets a tummy tuck. As a result, the presurgical marking may take longer since the surgeon will need to carefully position the skin in the place it will be after the surgery.

Set up an appointment with the plastic surgeon. Just as you did with the weight-loss surgery, it's a good idea to write your questions down before your appointment and jot down the surgeon's responses during your consultation. Also, be sure to bring your updated list of medications and supplements, as well as a list of your comorbidities. Comorbidities—particularly in the areas of heart, lungs, and blood pressure—must be considered in making a determination about whether plastic surgery is possible and whether you are a good surgical risk. Add to your list any problems you've had with anesthesia or prior surgeries. If you still smoke or have an alcohol problem, it is very important to be honest about it.

Plastic surgery is an elective surgery that can have profoundly positive effects both medically and psychologically. It is also serious surgery that can take from less than three hours to up to eight hours and, as with all surgeries, has significant risks including infection, lung problems, deep venous thrombosis, and pulmonary embolus. These postoperative complications can be reduced with preoperative antibiotics, good surgical technique, and close attention to wound care. Discuss what you expect from your surgery as well as the possible risks very thoroughly with your plastic surgeon before making your decision.

Many people have the mistaken notion that all of the tissue, fat, and skin areas can be corrected at once. This is not possible. Depending on your specific areas of concern, multiple surgeries may be necessary. Plastic surgery on the abdomen—in this case, abdominoplasty—is the most common surgery following weight-loss surgery. In this procedure, excess fat and skin are removed and excessively stretched, loose muscles are repaired. Hernias can also be repaired during abdominal surgery. Follow-up to the surgery is generally simple. People can usually return to work in about a month, and sometimes sooner. After complete healing from the abdominal surgery, breast and arm surgery can be considered. The aim of the breast surgery—including the insertion of a prosthesis, mastoplexy, or breast lift—is to create normal size and volume, and to reduce psychological distress caused by, in many instances, shapeless, flattened breasts that were previously full. Lessened sensation is rare and probably occurs in about 5 percent of the cases. Arm surgery is primarily for cosmetic reasons to reduce the excess skin on the upper arm. Body-lift surgery, which is the third step that a limited number of people choose, is a complete lift of the lower body. This procedure is more serious and may have greater risks. Scarring can be significant as the incision circles the entire body and may be extremely long. The abdomen, buttocks, hips, and thighs are all lifted at the same time. The recovery period may be a long one. The dramatic results of this surgery should be weighed against the risks and extended recovery time. Also available are thigh lifts that deal with excessive wrinkling, sagging, and bagginess of the thighs, and facelifts that deal with sagging of the facial skin.

Remember, plastic surgery is elective. Like all surgeries, it entails risks. In many cases it can also have profound positive physical and psychological effects. Weigh your decision carefully!

CONCLUSION

Hopefully what you discovered in this chapter is that you have not lost your best friend: You *are* your best friend. You haven't lost your identity; you are just redefining it. You are still *you* despite the major changes you're going through. You're learning not only to feel but also to value and express the feelings you have. You've put a stop to those destructive messages you had come to rely on and have replaced them with positive truths about yourself. There are new aspects to your identity that are just waiting to be explored! Without your heavy reliance on food, there's so much more space, time, and energy to become who you are meant to be and to develop long-lasting relationships with other people. You are looking and feeling so much better. This is a new and exciting time to be moving on! This is truly a second chance. Let's turn now to your relationships with others.

CHAPTER 12

ℋ SECOND CHANCE—
YOUR RELATIONSHIPS
WITH OTHERS

Your surgery and the months that followed may seem like a distant memory now. You're getting out and about in the world in a different way than you were before your surgery. With all the changes that have been taking place both inside and out, it's not surprising if you feel like you've been on an emotional roller coaster. Chances are, you've been finding these internal and external changes confusing and disorienting. Previous chapters have taken an in-depth look at what your body is going through, as well as some of the things that have taken place inside you. In this chapter, we'll take a look at the changes that might be taking place in your interpersonal relationships. This should help you navigate the sometimes tricky and possibly newly emerging world of intimacy.

The road to positive, lasting relationships—whether platonic or romantic—isn't always easy. In most cases, some old friendships, your marriage, your relationships with family members, and some of your dealings with coworkers and social acquaintances will undergo a transformation. You may be embarking on the world of dating for the first time in a long time. You'll also be making new friends. Success in all of these cases requires care and attention. Therefore, this chapter will arm you with some of the information you need to make your second chance with others the best that it can be.

HOW OTHERS PERCEIVE YOU NOW

With the positive changes in your appearance, you'll probably find that you are more confident and assertive in your dealings with other people. This should make it easier for you to develop new relationships and strengthen old ones. In fact, you're probably socializing more with new and old friends. There will, of course, be difficulties to overcome.

Most of the people who knew you before your surgery will see the dramatic difference in how you look. The physical changes, as well as the changes that have taken place inside you, may influence their perception of you. As for any new people you happen to meet, they won't judge you or have any preconceived notions of who you are based solely on your body weight. Believe it or not, how new people view you can sometimes be a bit complicated. They will be seeing you as the slimmer, happier, and healthier person you have become and won't know anything about your underlying past issues or the pain that may have played a role in your presurgical weight, nor will they know anything about the consequences your weight had on you. They will not know that echoes of these past issues may still remain and, at times, can cause unexplained sensitivities.

You may be quite surprised that people who didn't give you the time of day in the past stop to talk with you now. You may have been seeing the same familiar faces for years—at supermarkets, on your regular route to work, at your house of worship, and at school or work—but they had never approached you before, nor you them. Even if you are like some of our patients who don't want the attention or understandably remain rooted in anger at past hurts, try to enjoy the attention. You look and feel so much better, and it shows. This is what will shine through when people encounter you now. This is how they will perceive you. Try to take pleasure in it.

YOUR RELATIONSHIPS WITH YOUR OLD FRIENDS

If you took our advice in earlier chapters, you probably discussed your decision to have weight-loss surgery with your close friends. A few of these friends or one special one may have become an important part of your support system, accompanying you to meetings and appointments, asking questions, listening to your concerns, and reassuring you. Others may have lent their support simply by being available to chat or see a movie. Whatever the case, as you change, some of these friends—in some cases, even your most avid supporters—may suddenly become very distant and difficult to read. Some may be jealous of your success; others may begin to compete with you. In some cases, if you ask them to share their feelings with you, they may clam up. Others may be sarcastic or do or say hurtful things without warning. For example, after Kate had lost 150 pounds, her longtime roommate stunned her when she said she no longer wanted Kate to be a bridesmaid at her wedding. Kate says, "The fear of change is very real in many people. Friends want you to be a constant in their lives, just as you are. I think that when we decide to change—even for the better—we need to give our friends and our family as much support as we are asking for in return. Tell them it's okay to be angry with you—to be afraid of losing the old you. If the relationship is worth working on for you, it should be for them too. Some can't, or won't, grow with you; unfortunately, taking care of yourself might require that you restrict or sever that connection. But reach out that hand when you can, and you might end up the biggest winner of all." In another case, Randy's friends teased her about deserting them for the "150 Club," the name they'd made up for all of the people in the world who weighed 150 pounds or less. Randy was able to assure her friends that she would never desert them, and, in this case, she was able to close the distance before it was irreversible.

If you find one or more of your good friends behaving differently toward you in a way that makes you feel uncomfortable, try talking things through with them. Talking can help you get at the root of the problem and nip it in the bud before it blossoms into something bigger. Remember, you are the one who is changing, so in most cases, it is up to you to take the first step. In the rare case where this is not possible, move on. Keep in mind also that with your increased energy and physical health, you'll be wanting to try all the things you weren't able to do before—for example, traveling or engaging in sports or other physical activities. Some of your old friends may not be able to do these things with you because of physical limitations or simply may not be interested. In fact, your relationship with some of your old friends, maybe even your closest friend, may have been centered on eating. For example, Kristi's best friend of twenty-five years didn't speak to her for a month after the surgery. "She didn't even show up at the hospital," Kristi said. "I think she felt betrayed. When I told her I was having the surgery, she'd said to me, 'Does this mean we can't eat together?' I assured her that I'd still be able to eat, just not as much, and that I would still attend her parties and enjoy her food. I explained that eating would become an issue of quality, not quantity. She eventually came around and we're still best friends. She knows I'm the same person."

In some cases, you and your old "eating" partners, if they are close friends, may be able to come up with some creative ideas of how else you can spend your time together—for example, rent a movie, do craft projects, start a book club, try something new and adventurous, do something active, sit and talk, or share new approved recipes. If maintaining the friendship is important to both of you, you'll find a way to work it out and find new common interests.

It certainly takes a lot of courage to be honest about your feelings and to let your old friends know that you still value their presence in your life. Sometimes this will deepen your friendships. In other cases, sadly, you'll need to move on and develop friendships with others. In this case, it will be important for you to begin joining new groups and activities that you may have avoided in the past. There is a whole world out there filled with old friends and new caring people just waiting for you.

YOUR RELATIONSHIP WITH YOUR PARENTS AND/OR CHILDREN

Some parents are very supportive of their adult child's decision to have weight-loss surgery. They are fully aware of how obesity has limited their child's life and how it has affected their health; they are confident the surgery will make things better. Your parents may have been all for it when you told them you were thinking about the surgery. They probably know how hard it was for you to lose weight over the years. And, assuming you discussed things with them, they know how much thought you put into having the surgery and how much research you did. Even if your parents are difficult to deal with in general, chances are they have been and will remain supportive throughout your journey. Other parents, however, may not be able to give their support. They may fear for your safety, despite your assurances, or may think you're perfect just the way you are. Sometimes, they don't really know much about the surgery and educating them can help. If not, for this reason, some of our patients choose not to tell their parents and attribute their fantastic new look to diet.

In all cases, it is certainly up to you to decide who to tell about the surgery. But, if you can be honest with your parents, that's usually the best route to go. You may find their input comforting as you go through the postsurgical changes and challenges.

If you have children, they will probably be very proud of your weight-loss success. It's important to include them in what's going on with you. You are a model of what bravery, hard work, and determination can achieve. You'll also be serving as a model for healthy eating. Involve your children in shopping and planning for meals. This will help them share in your success. Also, you may find yourself right beside your kids, actively participating in some of the things you'd enjoyed only as a spectator in the past. Surely, they'll take great delight in this. Planning day excursions or

Setting a Good Example

The research linking genetics and obesity is becoming more solid, but we don't need science to know that if one family member is obese, other family members also tend to be obese. In addition, the husbands and wives of our obese patients frequently have significant weight problems, as well. When people realize, by example, that the surgery is not as frightening as they had feared and see the positive changes in their loved one, they often begin to consider surgery for themselves. For example, Vicki says, "My husband had the surgery three and a half years ago, when he weighed 520 pounds. When I met his surgeon, I felt like he was giving me the once-over for surgery. 'Anytime you're ready,' he said. I felt foolish. Later, we went to a party. None of the guests had seen my husband since the surgery. By then, he'd lost 200 pounds and was doing great. A lot of people asked me when I was going to have the surgery since his was such a success. The next day, I attended the support group. Now, I'm five weeks post-op and have lost forty-three pounds!"

longer trips to places you and the kids have dreamed of visiting will open up a new world for all of you. Most important, sharing your success with your children in this manner can create deeper bonds.

"My fifteen-year-old son is very proud of me," said Wendy. "He tells me how excited he is that I'm becoming smaller. I'm sure he's been embarrassed by my size, and that makes me sad. Now he's just happy that I'm healthy. He encourages me to keep up the good work and tells me how great I look. I think he's looking forward to having a 'super' mom!"

YOUR RELATIONSHIP WITH YOUR SPOUSE

The period following weight-loss surgery tends to make good marriages better and difficult marriages worse, sometimes ending in divorce. If you are married, what can you do to improve the odds? Start by expressing what's going on inside you so the changes don't come as a shock one day. Hopefully, your spouse has been beside you every step of the way. As you journey toward long-term health, try to help your spouse to be your best ally and friend—your partner in "forever health." Most of our patients' husbands or wives turn out to be very supportive and proud of their mates' successes, particularly if they've been attending their support groups.

All marriages are different, of course, but we've seen some similarities among our patients. If you're like many of our patients, you're probably very used to doing things for others. You may have been relatively passive in your marriage and asked your spouse for very little. This is because some morbidly obese people feel like they deserve very little. If this is where you're coming from, you may find that as you lose weight, you become more assertive and confident. You may begin to ask for more. If your spouse was used to being in control all of the time, she may be taken aback by your new needs and desires. Naturally, you'll want to be more in control of your own life now. You won't be content with someone else calling all of the shots any longer. You'll know that you deserve more and will want that much more out of life. Be sure to express to your spouse what's going on with you and work to create and maintain a new balance that works for both of you. Remember, this is a second chance. If you and your spouse can work together to anticipate and weather the changes that will occur, chances are you'll become closer than ever.

Unfortunately, however, as you lose your weight, a few of you may find that your spouse is becoming even more controlling out of fear that she will lose you. One husband was so frightened by the prospect of losing his wife that he tried to force-feed her large amounts ice cream! If your spouse is obese, she may feel like there's a competition going on between the two of you. Jealously can also be an issue now that you're getting more attention from people of the opposite sex, even if they're just friends. These feelings are not unusual and must be dealt with. If you have difficulty resolving these feelings on your own, consider seeing a psychotherapist or family counselor as soon as possible. If these things are not openly discussed, they can fester into suspicion, distrust, increased efforts at control, and, in the worst case, verbal or physical abuse. In more extreme cases, if you are being verbally or physically abused by your spouse, get immediate help. You are not worthless or undeserving, and you do not have to put up with such behavior—ever.

"After months of discussions with my husband, I announced my decision to go ahead with the surgery," Tina said. "He became so upset and said the only reason I wanted to have the surgery was so I could leave him and find someone better to marry. After the surgery, his jealousy escalated. I was shocked and hurt. Then, I became very angry. It was then that I realized how much emotional and verbal abuse I had been taking from him for so many years. Why had I ignored it? After a heated argument, he hit me for the first and last time. I called the police, and eventually we got divorced."

In some cases, morbidly obese patients didn't have much of an opportunity to date before marriage. Mingling with members of the opposite sex may not have been a big part of their lives. Sometimes the dating scene may have involved sexual or verbal abuse or just poor treatment. With that as a backdrop, some of our patients marry the first interested person, whether or not they would have been the first choice or even a good choice. They may feel that the person they chose to marry was all that they deserved. However, with the changes that take place after surgery, they start feeling better about themselves and delight in the attention they are getting from the opposite sex. If you recognize yourself in any of this, know that this period can be a potential disaster for your marriage. As your excitement in the wonderful changes you are experiencing grows, you may find yourself eager to experience all that you have missed. You may wonder why you married the person you did. You may feel a strong urge to just move on. This is not unusual. You will certainly be moving on to so many new things. However, the decision to leave your marriage deserves very serious thought. For some, the decision to divorce has been a long time in coming and is a positive step. For others, counseling may help to repair old hurts and create a new and more positive relationship.

ROMANTIC AND SEXUAL RELATIONSHIPS

If you are like many of our patients, you've spent a good deal of time imagining what it would be like to be thin. It's possible that these daydreams centered on finding Prince or Princess Charming and living happily ever after. Unfortunately, it's not that easy. Dating and finding the right mate can be an enormously difficult and complex process with lots of confusing twists and turns for anyone—whether obese or thin, atttractive or homely. "I dated off and on for a year," said Mindy. "Being new on the singles' scene at age thirty-six, I was warmly received. It surprised me that only confident, successful men asked me out for lunch and dinner. I was amazed by all the attention. Business cards were floating around my purse. It was just too much! I was overwhelmed and couldn't cope, so I put them all in a rubber band in the back of my dresser drawer and didn't respond to any of them."

In many cases, people who were obese as teenagers and young adults did not date much. In some cases, sexuality may have become synonymous with being used or abused. (See the inset "A History of Sexual Abuse" on page 227.) Having little chance to practice skills with the opposite sex or having negative sexual experiences can result in arrested social development. Because of this, some people may be afraid to take the plunge. Tim, a single man, told us, "My major concern about dating is my damaged self-image and my lack of social interaction with women. At more than three hundred forty pounds, I hadn't been on a date in sixteen years." Tim didn't know how to go about getting out there. He needed to work on repairing his self-image. And with the help, support, and encouragement of his support group, as well as his therapist, he began to broaden his social network, joining new activities, attending mixed social events, and dating again.

If you are just now entering the dating world, a lack of comfort and arrested socials skills with the opposite sex, as well as a damaged self-image, may cause you some reluctance to proceed. This can be an issue for you until you build up some self-confidence and have the opportunity to practice your social skills. On the other hand, you may be like some people who want to make up for lost time and can't wait to join the dating scene, seemingly without reservations. They know they look good and have a new respect for, and more confidence in, themselves. "I joined an Internet dating service two weeks ago," Cathy told us. "In the past, I'd experienced so much rudeness from men toward obese women that I used to shy away from dating. But now, I'm really looking forward to it, and I'm looking forward to finding a worthy companion!"

In some cases, sex and sexuality become key issues during this time. Some of our patients have worn their excess weight like a kind of protective shield. Now that the shield is down—in other words, the weight has come off—they suddenly feel very vulnerable. They may still feel uncomfortable with their bodies, despite the fact that they look better. In this case, their discomfort with their bodies probably has more to do with it than just excess weight. Here's what Erica said, "I sense that I should not push myself too hard, and so I gently nurture my sexual feelings, allowing them to progress at a slow pace. If I have used my weight in the past to avoid dealing with sexual issues, I worry that I might regress and try to regain weight if I feel exposed or vulnerable." It helps to discuss any fears and/or negative feelings you have regarding your sexuality with a therapist. She may be able to help you identify and overcome the cause.

Others find their new sexuality liberating. They feel good about how they look, how they feel, and their freedom of movement. "I'm much more agile, which is a good thing all around," Cathy told us. "I feel more able to express myself sexually and to be sure that I am fulfilled. I'm just sexier and more confident than I used to be. I'm also not as afraid to ask for what I need and want." Cathy's new confidence has given her an outlet for sexual fulfillment. She's no longer afraid to ask for what she wants and deserves. Likewise, Tina said, "Sex is a lot better after the weight loss. It's much more enjoyable. I'm more easily aroused and excited."

A History of Sexual Abuse

For some people, the prospect of becoming sexually active raises a traumatic red flag. Why is this? The reason lies more in the past than in the present. Nationwide, weight-loss surgery professionals are surprised by the number of morbidly obese people who report having been victims of childhood sexual abuse. Quite often, the ramifications and indeed the memories of past sexual traumas may resurface following massive weight loss, causing emotional and psychological problems that should be examined and resolved. Unfortunately, weight-loss surgery alone will not cure the deep-seated pain and emotional damage caused by childhood abuse. Psychotherapy, however, can help make major inroads into understanding and resolving these memories and feelings, allowing for fuller enjoyment of one's sexuality and one's life.

Dani, one of the many patients we've met who was abused as a child, told the following story at her support group. "When I look back on my childhood, I'm horrified. I can't remember when the physical and verbal abuse began," she said. "I must have been very young. When I turned ten, the abuse became sexual. I was so scared and depressed, but I said nothing, hoping that someone would notice the pain in my eyes and help me. No one did.

"When I was eleven, I discovered that food could help me detach and feel better. As I withdrew more and more into myself, food became love, affection, nurturance, and understanding. The abuse continued. So did the eating. I began to hate men, but more important, I began to hate myself. I ate my way through my teen years until I was practically numb. By the end of high school, I weighed 300 pounds."

When Dani told this story, she was surprised by how many people in the group could relate to her experience. For the first time in her life, she realized that she was not alone. And so began her path toward recovery. If you can relate to Dani's story, you're not alone either. Seek help, if you haven't already, so that you too can begin to recover from these past injustices.

These are just a few of the issues and thoughts that may be on your mind regarding dating and sexuality. The key to joining the dating scene and eventually becoming intimate is to take it slow. Join new activities and groups where the chances of meeting new people with similar interest are very good. You can even join a singles' or single parents' group if you'd like. Consider groups that center on quiet activities like art, music, books, or theater—or on active interests such as golf, skiing, hiking, bicycling, or sailing. A period of trial and error is not uncommon, so don't let it put you off. Try not to be surprised by the twists and turns. If a relationship doesn't blossom or go the way you want, you can certainly go in search of another. In any case, you're likely to have fun and develop many new friendships by becoming more socially active, whether or not you develop any romantic relationships. You are opening the door to a new and wonderful world. Be open to surprises—enjoy it!

YOUR PROFESSIONAL RELATIONSHIPS

Some people are very fortunate to work in a supportive environment with bosses and coworkers who have a strong sense of professionalism. On the whole, their obesity does not influence their jobs or their professional relationships. They're likely to get time off from work for surgery and recovery without a hassle, and are likely to be respected for their bravery and subsequent success. Cathy was one of these fortunate people. "My boss was great through the whole experience," she said. "He supported my decision to have the surgery and was there to listen to me when I was having trouble getting insurance approval. When the surgery was set, he willingly gave me the time off from work that I would need. When I returned to work, he continued to support and encourage me. Now I feel great. All of my coworkers and even the president of the company are constantly telling me how great I look and how proud they are of my success. This positive feedback from my colleagues adds so much to my self-confidence, and I'm sure it makes my job performance even better.

In any job where constant contact with the public is a must, morbid obesity can be a deciding factor in job assignments and promotions. Some of our patients who work in the area of sales felt that, because of their appearance and the image it projected, they were kept back from the front lines, important sales contacts, and meetings. For example, Linda was the most experienced and successful salesperson on her team. Many of her sales were made through phone contacts, while other people on her team got the frontline opportunities. It wasn't only Linda's appearance that held her back, but also her shyness and self-consciousness. Today, Linda is 130 pounds lighter; she's changed her hairstyle and has gotten a whole new wardrobe. With her increased energy and vitality, she's more assertive and self-confident. She's currently being sent out on all of the top sales calls and is even more successful than she was before.

Other people, like Patti, have intentionally held themselves back out of self-consciousness about their weight. Patti recalls, "I wasn't so receptive about going out on sales calls before I lost my weight. I spent a lot of time training in the company because it meant I didn't have to worry about presenting myself to the public—it was safe and the relationships were safe. Now that I've lost weight, I am more receptive to venturing outside of that safe area. In fact, my job is sending me out into the public more often. Being more attractive is a definite plus, and I feel really good about meeting new clients."

In some cases, being overweight prohibits a person from moving into a specific career even with the best qualifications and training. Before her surgery, Susan explained, "I earned two college degrees. I'm a commercial pilot and a flight instructor, but no commercial airline would hire me because of my weight." Despite her frustration, through drive and willpower, Susan made the best of the situation but problems with her weight still remained. "I reconciled myself to the fact that my career would not be in the cockpit and found a wonderful career in aviation. Four years and two promotions later, I have taken an opportunity that involves traveling every month. While this is a dream come true for a frustrated pilot, I dread these trips because there's no airline seat that fits me. I hide the seatbelts from the flight attendants so that they don't see that I can't fasten them. Many of these business trips include air shows and tradeshows and involve walking and standing, which is excruciatingly painful for me. Obesity has shortchanged my career in other ways too. I have deferred many of my duties to an assistant who has the energy that I don't have even though it has hurt my standing in the company and jeopardized my chances for future promotions and favorable reviews."

Today, Susan is two years post-op. She, too, is confident and happy. She flies often and is at the forefront of her tradeshows. With her increased energy and absence of pain, she has taken over even more responsibility than before. She has been given the promotion she had been passed over for in the past. This is one of our many happy-ending stories, but despite an excellent new job after her surgery Susan found to her delight and surprise "other interests" becoming front and center—she became a mother!

CONCLUSION

The world is suddenly new and exciting, isn't it? You may find that you have new friends who share your growing interests and that you've developed deeper relationships with family members and old friends. Maybe you decided to end destructive relationships in favor of more fulfilling ones. Good for you! Your love life may be blossoming or maybe you're still working up the courage to get out and about. Whatever the case, try to spend as much time as you can with people who validate you and make you feel good about yourself. You have always been deserving of love and support. Go ahead and ask for it now, even if you're not used to doing so. Even more important, feel good about yourself! You deserve it!

PART FOUR

For Friends and Family

CHAPTER 13

$\mathcal{H}$OW YOU CAN MAKE A DIFFERENCE BEFORE SURGERY

I f you're reading this part, someone you care about is going to have weight-loss surgery. In this chapter and the next, we'll call this person your "loved one." This term can stand for many types of relationships.

You should feel proud to have been taken into this person's confidences. You've probably been an essential part of the process almost from the moment the idea to have surgery entered his mind. What can you do? Start by being there. Weight-loss surgery is a life-changing event that will have a profound effect on everyone who is close to this person. Throughout the presurgical process, as well as the days and weeks following surgery, you may be called upon to help in ways you might not have anticipated. The course your loved one has chosen can be surprisingly confusing and rocky. Although you may not have realized it, you may also need help. Therefore, this chapter and the chapter that follows are designed to help you provide the best care and support you can. You can be one person, hopefully among many, who helps make the difference between long-term success and failure.

BECOME INFORMED

Your first and most important task is to become informed along with the person facing surgery. You are already reading this book, and so have already begun the journey. Do your research to learn all you can about the various surgical procedures, the different surgeons, and the presurgical and postsurgical procedures and programs. Find out what you can from people who have been through the procedure. Listen to what their families have to say. They might be able to provide you with some important insight into what you're about to face as a support person. There is a great deal of information out there, and you should be able to find answers to any questions you might have. The Resources section lists some useful websites. If you choose to surf the Internet for information, see the inset "Sorting Out the Good From the Bad on the Internet" on page 90 for some useful advice. Don't forget that the surgeon's office will be available for any additional help or advice you might need. It can also provide you with sources of reliable information.

HELP KEEP THINGS ORGANIZED

Your loved one probably has a great deal of literature concerning weight-loss surgery. At times the sheer volume of information can be overwhelming. This is the perfect opportunity to give your loved one a presurgical gift—a large three-ring binder. Try to find one that's bright and colorful or decorate it yourself or with help from others. Get tabbed divider pages, and perhaps perforated folders, that fit into the binder. Some one-subject notebooks can also be clipped into the binder for note taking. These things will do wonders for keeping all the information neat and organized.

All of the accumulated information—for example, notes, handouts, copies of correspondence, doctors' reports, questionnaires, insurance information, instructions, and names and phone numbers of important people—will go into this binder. There can even be sections on helpful tips and questions to ask. With your loved one's permission, add any information that you think may be helpful. For example, you might want to put together a list of services—such as groceries stores that deliver, child-care workers, cleaning services, and so on—that your loved one can turn to after surgery. Include the names and address of important support group members, as well as any literature received at the support-group meetings.

This binder will certainly be a useful and thoughtful gift. Not only will it be an important source of information, but it will also serve as a source of comfort and strength throughout the entire process. This gift also benefits you. Since you'll probably be feeling anxious about the whole process yourself, this project will give you the opportunity to channel that somewhat nervous energy in a constructive and useful manner.

ACCOMPANY YOUR LOVED ONE TO MEDICAL APPOINTMENTS

If you've read Chapter 6, you have a pretty good idea of what will occur during the first visit to the weight-loss surgeon's office. It's natural and normal for your loved one to be experiencing a wide range of strong emotions—from fear and desperation to elation and anticipation. You can serve as an anchor, helping him to remain calm, clearheaded, and focused on the issues at hand. It's not uncommon for people facing surgery to feel anxious, and since anxiety can interfere with memory, you'll need to listen carefully to everything you hear to fill in the blanks later on. Don't be afraid to take notes of your own; carry a small pad and pencil in your pocket. It's essential that you try not to take over, but don't be afraid to ask any questions on your mind or remind your loved one of the questions he wanted to ask. In some cases, you may want to compile a list of questions together prior to the office visits.

GO WITH YOUR LOVED ONE TO THE SUPPORT GROUP

If you've been given the opportunity to accompany your loved one to a support-group meeting, do take advantage of it. Your presence there will benefit both of you. You'll find an invaluable source of information available to you at these meetings. Patients' testimonials, the surgeon's lectures, experts, and guest speakers usually cover a wide variety of interesting and informative topics. You'll have a chance to ask questions and meet other support people like yourself. In time, some may even become lifelong friends.

It's perfectly natural for you to be anxious, and perhaps somewhat ambivalent, about the surgery; therefore, another benefit of attending the support group is the chance to meet people who've had the surgery. Hearing how it has positively affected their health and lives will reassure you by helping you develop a better understanding of your loved one's choice.

Jenny tells how her support group helped alleviate some of her husband's reservations: "Even though my husband had attended the first meeting with me and got answers to many of his questions, he was still very unsure about my decision. At the next meeting he attended with me, he expressed concern about how I would eat after the surgery. He was invited to join the group for dinner following the meeting. He was surprised to see that the members seemed to be eating much more normally than he expected. He also noted how vibrant, healthy, animated, and energetic everyone seemed to be. They seemed to take joy in being together and in being alive. Later, back at home, he told me how glad he was that he had dinner with the group—everyone, he said, was so friendly, but more important, they seemed happy and healthy. And that, he said with excitement in his voice, is what he wants for me. Aren't I lucky?"

HELP MAKE THE FINAL DECISION

Deciding whether or not to have weight-loss surgery is one of the most important decisions a person will ever have to make. Virtually anyone who knows that there's a choice to be made will offer his opinion about the best course to follow. Some will be educated opinions, and others will be based on ignorance or fear. It's important to help your loved one figure out where these people are coming from and if their opinion should be taken into consideration.

The very important reality is that this is a very personal decision and, ultimately, must be made by your loved one alone. However, there are some things you can do to help. First and most important, with your loved one's permission, help sort out fact from fiction. Reexamine all of the accumulated information no matter how many times the two of you have gone through it. Next, help your loved one make a list of pros and cons, and go over them together. Be sure to listen, listen, listen. Try to fully and completely understand your loved one's point of view. Talk about what you feel, but don't be pushy.

Suggest that your loved one create a dream, or wish, list. This can include all those things your loved one dreams of as a thin person. This tends to be highly personal information so reserve your judgment, listen carefully, and express curiosity if appropriate. Go over the list together. This will not only help your loved one make the decision, but will certainly deepen your understanding of him. You can also be helpful in exploring the path your loved one must take in making these dreams a reality.

Always remember that the ultimate decision isn't yours to make. In the end, it is essential that you respect and support the final decision. You know full well that arriving at this place hasn't been easy. Reassure your loved one that you will be there no matter what happens.

BE THE "GO-BETWEEN"

At times throughout the process, you will likely be the person people turn to with questions they are too afraid to ask the person facing surgery. If you cannot answer their questions, make a note of them and try to find the answers. If you feel the questions are inappropriate, gently let them know that the information is private. Also, be aware that you—not the person considering the operation—may often be besieged with opinions about the surgery, some of which may be very strong. At times, people who approach you about your loved one's decision may seem irrational or extremely negative or even biased, and perhaps full of misinformation. Whenever possible, your task is to gently correct them by sharing the facts that you know to be true. In more extreme cases, you may need to protect your loved one from the onslaught of negative, although well-intentioned, opinions that aren't based on fact but, rather, appeal to irrational levels of fear and anxiety. Kristi gives this example: "My husband was with me every step of the way during the learning process," she told us. "When my family members were in disagreement about the surgery, he defended my choice. He reassured them that I was in need of a healthier life and that surgery would help me achieve that goal. He defended my choice to take such serious measures and assured my family that I would never do something like this if I didn't think it would save my life. This was a tremendous help!"

ASSIST IN THE PREPARATIONS FOR SURGERY

Once the decision has been made to have the operation, your loved one will begin the presurgical journey. At times, this journey can be quite complicated. You and other caring friends and family members can help smooth the path. Whenever possible, children should be involved in presurgical preparations. This will help make the upcoming events seem more natural and should help allay their fears somewhat by providing them with concrete tasks.

On a physical level, it's useful for people scheduled for weight-loss surgery to prepare for the life changes they must make after the surgery by incorporating new and healthier habits into their everyday routines well before the surgery takes place. In fact, studies show that a positive postsurgical outcome is dramatically increased by presurgical preparations that include the addition of exercise and early nutritional changes. You should, therefore, try to motivate your loved one to make these changes; you can even participate in them now that the surgery is imminent. Other presurgical preparations will also be necessary, some of which are more involved than others. Exercise, nutritional changes, and other important presurgical matters are discussed in the sections that follow.

Help With a Presurgical Exercise Routine

When the surgery is over, regular exercise will be an integral part of your loved one's long-term weight-loss program. You'll probably find that you have also become more active after your loved one has the surgery. There will be so much more you can do together. In the meantime, it's important for your loved one to begin the habit of daily exercise whenever possible.

You can help make this transition to a more active lifestyle easier by participating in the exercises. Since people are more likely to maintain an exercise program when they have an exercise buddy, go ahead and take on this role. You'll be surprised at how quickly your own health and energy increase.

Exercise doesn't have to be strenuous: any enjoyable physical movement has value. You might want to start by taking daily walks together— you don't have to walk far. If joint pain, breathing difficulties, or any other comorbidities are a problem, as they are for many morbidly obese people, your loved one should get permission or exercise guidelines from his surgeon.

"Water walking"—that is, wading through water—is easier on the joints and is a good form of exercise. If a private pool or community pool is available to you, you may want to encourage this form of exercise. If wearing a bathing suit makes your loved one uncomfortable, consider making your visit to the community pool on off hours when it will be virtually empty. Also, splashing around in the pool is a fun activity to share with children. In addition to providing an excellent way to exercise, water walking and, of course, splashing can be a fun and memorable family activity. Moreover, the relaxing and healing powers of water will reduce everyone's tension and anxiety, which are not uncommon during the presurgical time.

Whatever exercise your loved one chooses or is instructed to do, go ahead and join in the activity regularly. It'll make it so much more pleasurable to exercise if company is available, and in the process you too will become healthier.

Help With Presurgical Nutritional Changes

It's important to implement certain nutritional changes prior to surgery. It's enormously helpful when friends and family members become involved in this process. The more involved family members are, the better the chances are of your loved one's long-term weight-loss success. Everyone should be familiar with the surgical program's postsurgical dietary regulations well before the surgery takes place. Although this book provides nutrition guidance of a general nature, more specific information should be available in the literature your loved one receives from the surgeon.

To make a fresh start, help clear out the kitchen of all trigger foods and any unhealthy foods. Then, help your loved one think of ways to improve old shopping and cooking habits. The task of searching for and trying creative recipes can be quite fun. Kids will enjoy coming up with healthy-eating ideas. In the process, everyone will learn more about what makes his or

---

Do You Want a Hard-Boiled Egg With That?

These days, many people are used to living on a fast-food diet. This may be true for your loved one. Assure him that although he will be giving up unhealthy, fattening fast food, he doesn't have to give up "fast food" entirely. Foods that require little preparation include protein shakes, precooked chicken strips, string cheese, yogurt, cottage cheese, and shelled hard-boiled eggs. These can be your loved one's new, healthier "fast food."

---

her body all that it can be. (See also Chapter 14 for some tips on helping to make your loved one's new eating style work after surgery.)

Make Arrangements for Help and Support After the Surgery

It's essential that your loved one get adequate rest and relaxation in the days prior to surgery. Being harried, stressed out, and anxious right before surgery will surely hinder recovery. Therefore, try to take on as many of the presurgical tasks as you can. However, keep in mind that you should not run yourself ragged. If you will be the caretaker after surgery, you'll need to reserve some of your energy and concentrate on pacing yourself rather than attempting to do everything in a rush. Some people heal more slowly than others, so it pays to plan ahead in order to be prepared for anything that may arise. There are many things you can do now to make the post-surgical time easier on everyone, including yourself. (Chapters 7 and 8 will give you some idea what tasks will be necessary before and after surgery.)

Although your loved one may not be accustomed to asking for help and support, now is the time to try a different approach. Put together a list of people who are willing to be on call or who have volunteered for specific tasks, such as preparing approved meals, straightening up, grocery shopping for healthy foods, or even lifting heavy items if necessary. You'll find that most people will be happy to be assigned a task, and their help will prove to be a wonderful support.

Reassure Children

How children react to the whole presurgical process depends a lot on how old they are. No matter the age, however, the events leading up to the surgery will be scary and confusing. After all, their parent is facing a major challenge. During this stressful time, it's easy for them to get "lost in the

Get-Well Gifts

Although they mean well, some people may offer your loved one unapproved foods, such as candy, as part of their get-well gift. Such prepackaged, potentially harmful gifts should obviously be avoided. Other people may actually bring cakes and pies or send platters of cookies, which may be customary for some ethnic groups. Before this becomes an issue, remind people in the weeks prior to the surgery that your loved has certain nutritional requirements now and can no longer eat certain foods. If someone wishes to send a gift, suggest flowers, pillow spray, magazines, or videos. The best gift of all, however, is the gift of time.

shuffle." Even if they are not your children, you can still do a lot to support and reassure them.

You may want to help your loved one come up with ways to explain to small children what's going on. For example, one patient told her child, "I am going into the hospital to fix my insides and make me better. You will not see me for a few days, but I'll be home before you know it. Then, we'll be together. Daddy and your brother will stay with you at the house while I am in the hospital." True, but simple.

It might be a good idea for older children to attend a support-group meeting. Perhaps they can speak with the surgeon's office staff about what to expect before and after surgery. With smaller children, a simple handshake and a smile from the surgeon "who will be taking such good care of his or her mommy or daddy" may do wonders for their comfort level. Speak freely with older children about what's going on. Answer their questions simply and clearly. You don't need to provide more information than they ask for.

If you are one of the parents, it's important to be aware that you're going to be very busy for at least a week when your loved one gets home from the hospital. Although you may be used to taking care of the kids, you're probably going to need some help. When your friends or family members ask what they can do, this is it! Even if you'll be home full time during your loved one's recovery, try to make arrangements for people to spend quality time with your children or to help out with their basic needs. Still, you might find that caring for some of their basic needs on your own is a comfort during this stressful time. It's a good idea to notify your children's teachers that a parent will be in the hospital. This way, the teacher can better understand and deal with any changes in behavior, which are not unusual during times like these. In addition, he can provide the child with a little extra attention in the classroom.

Be sure to remind your children that their mom or dad will be getting better every day and that he will be moving toward much better long-term health. Most important, although many thing will be going on, try to make things as normal as possible for the children. When it comes to kids, normalcy is key.

Other Presurgical Matters

The simple tasks of getting things in order include cleaning the house, buying groceries, arranging for child care, and doing yard work. Also, it's important to make sure that the family car is running well in case of an emergency. Some people want to update their wills before going in for surgery or may want to prepare a living will as discussed in Chapter 7. Be sure the will or living will is handy and accessible. Likewise, all-important paperwork, such as life, medical, and disability insurance documents, should be accessible if needed. Also, go over any work-related matters with your loved one. Find out what to do if a coworker should call or if there is some sort of office emergency. Get the names of coworkers or supervisors who will need to be contacted in case of complications.

Additionally, you'll want to make the home as inviting and comfortable as you can for your loved one's return. This may include things like buying extra pillows or arranging for a hospital bed. Think about what would make your loved one's homecoming special. Get kids involved in the plans.

As you are now aware, there are many things to take care of in the weeks and days before surgery. Most of these things were discussed in Chapter 7. Copy the checklist in that chapter and help your loved one cover all of the bases.

SEEK EMOTIONAL SUPPORT FOR YOURSELF

Your loved one is going to be relying very heavily on you for a time. In order for you to provide the support he needs, you'll need to take care of yourself too. You may feel pressured and overwhelmed by all of the information and preparation. Also, although you know that the odds of success are in your loved one's favor, particularly with the lower risks in recent years, you know that there's the possibility of complications, which are sometimes life threatening. With all this going on, you may find that your emotions are all over the place. This is completely normal. As a support person, you'll be expected to remain strong for your loved one and any children involved. Therefore, there will be times when you too need support from someone you trust. This person may be another member of the family, a close friend, a religious/spiritual advisor, a therapist, someone you met at the weight-loss-surgery support group, or, for some, a higher power.

Although most people undergoing weight-loss surgery expect a positive outcome, there are times when this does not occur. This is not the norm, of course, but it will prove to be the moment that tries every ounce of your endurance and strength. It is also the time when you are the most in need of support to just get through. For example, Gina was at her husband David's side from day one—she attended the support group, accompanied him to medical visits, and helped him arrive at an informed decision. They hoped for and expected the best, but David had an unexpected postsurgical medical crisis. Without family and friends close by, Gina found comfort in communicating with them on a daily basis via the Internet. She was able to share with them David's progress as well as her own stresses and frustrations. When David was recovering, he, too, found the Internet messages extremely comforting. David is fine now, by the way, at half the size he was before the surgery.

CONCLUSION

This chapter has given you some idea of what is expected of you as a support person in the months, weeks, and days leading to your loved one's surgery. The next chapter will give you some idea of what to expect during the recovery period, and once again, how you can be an integral part of your loved one's long-term surgical success.

CHAPTER 14

$\mathcal{A}$FTER SURGERY, YOU ARE ESSENTIAL

After what may have seemed like a never-ending wait, the surgery is finally over. The months of uncertainty, fear, excitement, and anticipation are behind you. The surgery may have left your loved one feeling weak and looking a bit pale, but she has most likely come through the procedure with flying colors. Now that you've gotten through the worst of it, the path ahead will be easier, or so you assume. Don't lull yourself into thinking this. Sure, you can relax and breathe a sigh of relief now that the surgery is over, but there's still more, much more, to your loved one's journey, and you can help.

You are keenly aware of the fact that for many years or even decades, your loved one has fought the weight-loss battle with no success. On all levels, you know in your mind and heart that this time the battle is very different. You fully and completely understand the severity of what's occurred and what's to come. Chances are you also attended support-group meetings and learned all the facts alongside your loved one. You've probably talked and talked about the surgery. You are knowledgeable and motivated. Unfortunately, that does not guarantee success. The most critical time is now, and, no matter how strong a person your loved one is, this is the time she will need you most. The key is to just be there.

This chapter is for you, for all of you, who wish to provide additional help and support throughout your loved one's recovery and subsequent weight loss. Being there will also help fuse and later strengthen your friendship or partnership. Working together will move you, your family and/or your extended family, and your loved one toward long-term "forever" health. Good luck!

AFTER THE SURGERY

It's finally over and now you're anxious to see your loved one. It's likely that after the surgery your loved one will be moved to a recovery room or the intensive-care unit. If you are permitted to see her at this point, don't be alarmed by what you see. The tubes, wires, IV lines, medical equipment, and so on are normal parts of the postsurgical process. To familiarize yourself with the types of things you might encounter, read the section "What the Tubes and Wires Are All About" in Chapter 8. The best thing you can do at this point is just be there. In fact, if you can be there when your loved one opens her eyes, that will be the best medicine.

Remember, it's normal for your loved one to look pale and weak after surgery, and it's also normal for her to be experiencing pain for the first few days after surgery, even with pain medication. Moreover, it's not uncommon for your loved one to be very, very tired—perhaps more tired than she has ever felt. Again, this is normal. Rest is essential for healing. (To help make sure your loved one gets the needed rest following surgery, see the inset "Swarms of Well-Wishers?" on page 245.)

There are many things that will be asked of you in the days to come. Read on to learn how you can help by reassuring children, dealing with doubts and fears, decorating the hospital room, and being your loved one's advocate with the nursing staff.

Reassure Children Once Again

Children will naturally want to see their mother or father as soon as possible after the surgery. How they react will depend largely on how you and other adults react, so try to remain calm. Avoid information overload. Children will tell you what they need to know by asking questions. Your response will, of course, depend on the age of the child, but answer questions as briefly and as simply as possible in a reassuring manner. In the case of children who are too young to see their parent immediately after surgery, a brief phone call when the patient is able to make one will go along way in assuring them that their mom or dad is getting better.

Help Deal With the Question "What Have I Done?"

When your loved one is moved into her regular room and has had some time to think, it's likely that the enormity of her new life situation will hit her. She may express fear and doubt. It's not uncommon for people who've had this surgery to ask, "What have I done?" In many cases, feeling fearful

Swarms of Well-Wishers?

We should all be lucky enough to have swarms of well-wishers wanting to see us after surgery! It's a great gift to have so many people who care. However, when many people (or even just a few) descend on your loved one at once so soon after surgery, you may need to serve as "tactful" gatekeeper for a while. Tell your loved one that people have come to visit, and if she is too tired to see them, let the visitors know how much you appreciate their coming, but that for now, rest is essential and visits must be limited. Suggest that they send cards, small gifts, flowers, and the like that your loved one can enjoy while in the hospital. Don't forget to remind well-wishers not to send candy, cake, cookies, alcohol, or similar food gifts. One light-hearted patient we know requested that visitors bring her books: "These books serve two purposes," she said with a smile. "I can read them when I get bored—or throw them at people when I want to be left alone!"

or doubtful after surgery is normal. You can help allay these feelings. For example, Jeanne, a weight-loss-surgery program director, says she hears this question all the time. She usually responds with a quick reality check: "Are you the same person who worked so hard to get insurance coverage and to schedule your surgery as soon as possible?" As a follow-up to this question, Jeanne says she'll usually show the post-surgical patient her letter to the insurance company, stating all the reasons she needed the surgery. This is a great answer to the question "What have I done?" Being reminded of all the reasons your loved one wanted the surgery can be incredibly therapeutic. So, it's a good idea to have your loved one's insurance letter handy. Better yet, bring the entire information binder with you; the insurance letter should be in there.

Provide Love and Affirmation

Love and affirmation are essential during what may be a very scary time for your loved one. Be positive and keep any negative thoughts and feelings at bay. Your loved one will feel very special if you decorate the room with visitors' cards and gifts as well as her positive affirmation posters (see page 132 in Chapter 8). In fact, before your loved one is moved into her hospital room, get permission from the nursing staff to decorate the room with the posters and any flowers or cards that have arrived. This will help raise your loved one's spirits more than you can imagine. (If the hospital stay will be very brief, consider decorating the room at home.)

Be Your Loved One's Advocate and Help Out in the Hospital

In many hospitals, the nursing staff has an overwhelming workload, with many more patients to look after than they had in the past. Therefore, it's important for you to be your loved one's advocate. Don't be afraid to ask questions, and if anything seems out of order, be sure to point it out! Also, ask the nursing staff how you can supplement the care they're giving your loved one.

As discussed in Chapter 8, your loved one will need to get up and walk around as soon as possible after surgery. Check with the staff on the appropriate times for exercise. During these times, you'll need to encourage your loved one to get up and walk even if she doesn't feel like it. She may feel like Cathy did: "After surgery all I wanted was to take my pain medication, curl up in a ball, and sleep." While these feelings are not uncommon, it's important not to give in to them. Therefore, encourage your loved one to take a walk to the bathroom, walk down the hall, or, at the very least, walk in place beside the bed with your support.

You can also help your loved one with her all-important breathing and leg-pumping exercises. These exercises will help her build strength, fend off complications, and speed recovery. Also, encourage your loved one to listen to her inspirational audiotapes. Hearing positive affirmations several times a day after surgery has proven to be incredibly helpful with improving self-image, lifting one's mood, and, in some cases, fending off the depression that may occur.

If you haven't already read Chapter 8, read it now. It will fill you in on many of the important happenings during your loved one's stay at the hospital. It should give you more ideas about how you can help care for her.

AT LONG LAST, THE RETURN HOME

No matter how brief the hospital stay, it may have seemed like forever. Now that your loved one is back at home, you'll probably want things to return to normal as soon as possible. You'll need to give it some time, however. We usually ask our post-surgical patients to behave at home in much the same manner they did in the hospital for a while. The approximate length of time to do this depends on the particular patient and the type of surgery she had. Your loved one's surgeon should be able to give you some idea how long this "hospital-like" behavior should continue.

There are many things your loved one will be unable to do for a while, so your continued help will be necessary. Erica, a strong and independent woman, summed it all up when she said, "After my surgery, my husband was wonderful. He completely relieved me of all responsibility. He got me what I needed to eat and drink, cleaned the house, went shopping, answered the phone, took me to medical visits, took care of the kids and the pets, and was totally supportive of my new way of eating. He even stopped eating fried foods! I felt like a queen!"

If you're anything like Erica's husband, you'll want to make your loved one's homecoming and the weeks ahead as comfortable and stress-free as possible. You'll also need to play an important part in reminding your loved one to follow all of the necessary steps and medical advice to ensure a complete recovery.

From reminders to eat and drink and keeping house to calling on friends for help and caring for kids—there will be lots for you to do. These things are discussed in the sections to follow.

Provide Round-the-Clock Care

Your loved one should not be left alone in the house even for brief periods at first, although this depends significantly on the type of surgery she had. If the surgeon recommends it (be sure to ask), someone should always be available to help with whatever she needs, especially in case of an emergency. Therefore, if you cannot be there, arrange for an adult to be available in the home at all times during the early recovery period. If friends or family members are not available for round-the-clock care, call a local community center, church, or the hospital to arrange for a homecare worker. Sometimes members of the support group can help with this task. (This, of course, should be arranged in advance.)

Remind Your Loved One to Eat and Drink

After surgery, your loved one may not feel hungry or thirsty. This will like be a new phenomena for both of you. However, it's very important for her to eat and drink at regular intervals. Our colleague Jarol B. Knowles, MD, MPH, of Duke University Medical Center, suggests that her patients use a timer to remind them to eat and drink at regular intervals. (A kitchen timer or a watch with an alarm can make a great postsurgical gift.) You can help set and monitor the timer, and then make sure that eating and drinking occur at these regular intervals. With your help, your loved one won't have to worry about waiting too long between meals.

Provide Creature Comforts

Comfort is essential when your loved one returns home from the hospital. If you've taken our advice, the house should be in good order. This, of course, is great news, because as caretaker, you'll have little time for chores for the next few weeks. After all, with all you've been through, you'll probably feel physically and emotionally tired, too. Therefore, be sure to prepare things beforehand. Have the room your loved one will be staying in made up, free of clutter (for ease of movement), and cheerfully decorated. Also, have extra sets of fresh sheets available for the bed or recliner, some fresh-scented pillow spray (to get rid of the hospital smell), extra pillows (for propping and coughing), a foot stool (for helping to get in and out of bed), and so on.

Call on Friends and Family

No matter how strong and capable you are, you can't expect to be able to do everything alone. You need your rest too! So now is the time to call on any willing friends and relatives for help. If there's something you've forgotten or need to take care of, don't hesitate to ask someone to take care of it for you. Quite often, people forget that caretakers also need support. Don't be afraid to remind them how much you would appreciate help. Helping out could simply involve coming over to stay with your loved one while you take a nap. Or it may involve bringing over approved foods if you run short on certain things.

Care for the Children and Child-Related Matters

Even if you're used to caring for the kids all the time, you may need some help in this area too. Once again, don't be afraid to call on people for assistance. Helping with the children can involve anything from preparing their lunches for a week or so, helping with homework, and taking them to school to dropping them off and picking them up from activities. Since eating at home will be a very different experience for now, you even might want to suggest that friends or relatives take the kids out to dinner. The movies, the park, or other fun places are also options. See if you can arrange play dates and sleepovers at friends' houses for the kids; this will give both you and your loved one time to rest.

Of course, some children will be afraid to let their parent out of their sight. For the first few days, it's perfectly natural for children to want to be as close to their recovering parent as possible. Although steps were probably taken to mentally prepare the kids, it's still frightening for them to see mom or dad in a weakened state. You'll need to be strong and in charge for their sake. Let the kids know that their parent is getting the best of care.

Once again, after the initial period, try to keep the kids busy with activities with many different people who care about them. The key for children, psychologically speaking, is to maintain their regular routines and activities as much as possible. Urge them to go to school and participate in their normal activities. Assure them that there is absolutely nothing wrong with participating in outside activities and having fun during their parent's recovery period. Remind them that their mom or dad will be improving each day and of all the positive ways family life will improve as they move together toward long-term health.

Be sure to remind your loved one of what a good parent she is and how it's okay during this time to rely on other people to help with the children. Since she may have little energy for a while, it shouldn't be too difficult to convince her not to try to be "superparent" for a while. Assure your loved one that just because she doesn't have mental or physical energy for the kids right now, it doesn't mean she is a "bad" parent.

By the way, it's a good idea to get in touch with the kids' teachers to let them know what's going on at home. The teachers may be willing to provide extra care and attention during this time and should understand that it may be difficult for the kids to concentrate on schoolwork or that their behavior may change.

Understand Mood Swings

Your loved one may be taking medication, which can affect her behavior. Also, tiredness, pain, and discomfort have a way of making people feel cranky. And, particularly in the case of women, the postsurgical spikes in estrogen levels may have their moods swinging from one extreme to the other—fear, courage, regret, anticipation, sadness, elation, and a variety of others, some of which may be indescribable. Additionally, as anesthesia leaves one's system, it can cause depression, even weeks after surgery. One patient we know referred to this time of her life as the worst case of PMS ever. The mood shifts can be so extreme that your loved one thinks she is going crazy. You might think so too! First and foremost, know that your loved one is *not* going crazy and assure her of that fact. This is probably a very temporary hormonally and chemically induced state. However, the surgeon should be made aware of this since medications are readily available to help.

Of all of these emotional states, depression can be particularly confusing. Although it may be, in part, a result of hormonal and chemical changes, other things may be going on inside to bring about these feelings. For example, Gina told us that her husband, David, was particularly weepy in the weeks following surgery. Although he went ahead with the surgery, he'd always denied that his weight was a problem (as many obese people do). After surgery, however, he could no longer deny how dangerous his condition had been. He found himself dwelling on the fact that he could have died as a result of his weight. He deeply regretted how his weight had limited every aspect of his family's life for so many years.

Gina's job was to listen, and that will be your job too. She supported and affirmed David's feelings. She even wept along with him when the feeling came over her. Then, she felt herself becoming angry. She explained to David in a very gentle way how his denial had affected her and their family. She'd held it in for so long that it felt good and therapeutic to let it out. She needed to talk honestly about her anger, and chances are you may too. Be gentle and caring and let your loved one know just how much you love her and appreciate what she has gone through to make a better life for all of you. Gina did this, and she and David were able to look toward their promising future. Today, all of that seems very far behind them, but it needed to happen, just as it may need to happen for you and your loved one. Resolve the past, but don't dwell excessively on it, and move toward the future.

Help Make the New Eating Plan Work

For as long as you can remember, food has probably been your loved one's friend and source of comfort, as well as her worst enemy. Eating styles and habits have surely become deeply ingrained in your loved one's life, and in many cases, in the life of the whole family and/or circle of friends. But all this must change! It's important for you to respect and appreciate how difficult this change can be.

More than anything else, it's essential to keep in mind that your loved one is completely aware of what she must do to fully comply with her new eating plan. It is absolutely essential that you also keep in mind that your loved one is solely responsible for that compliance. Do not under any circumstances tell them what to eat or drink. They already know what they should do and your reminder, no matter how kindly intended, may trigger a negative response. That said, there are some things you and others can do to make compliance with the new eating plan a whole lot easier.

Reduce Temptation

Remember, the purpose of weight-loss surgery is to help control the amount of food consumed and absorbed; it cannot eradicate the disease of obesity or the tendency to eat whatever and whenever to excess. This tendency may always lurk somewhere beneath the surface for the life of your loved one. One important thing you can do is to help reduce the temptation to eat unapproved foods by keeping sweets, junk food, and "binge foods" out of sight and well hidden. In fact, it's best to not keep these foods in the house at all. In many cases, people who compulsively overeat become masters at not only hiding food but also finding hidden food. In other words, it is highly unlikely that you'll be able to keep food hidden for any length of time. Therefore, if people who live in the house must eat sweets, junk food, and other types of foods that are not permitted, it's best to bring only small portions into the home at a time and eat these foods out of sight of your loved one.

Also, be aware that food smells, pictures of food, and discussions about food can trigger cravings—even after significant weight loss has occurred. For a while after the surgery, your loved one will likely experience few food cravings, lulling everyone into a false sense of security that they are gone forever. Unfortunately, as mentioned previously, food cravings can return with a vengeance about twelve to eighteen months after surgery. This is entirely normal, although it can be troublesome and disappointing. During this high-risk period for weight regain, you can help by remembering that "out of sight out of mind" is the order of the day.

Make Family-Wide Changes

When we suggest removing all junk food and sweets from the home, we often hear, "But what about the rest of the family? What about the kids?" Here's how we answer those questions: No one needs junk food to survive. Your loved one's new healthy eating habits can be the start of healthier eating for the whole family, and as a result, everyone will benefit! A new way of eating for everyone in the household can be especially helpful if other members of the family also have weight issues.

Make the move toward healthy eating habits a family-wide endeavor in the most positive sense. Search for new, healthy, and delicious recipes together and include children in the preparation. This simple task will help kids feel more included in what's going on. It will also help normalize what may seem like a confusing and distancing event.

Approach new foods with a sense of humor. Some of it will be quite tasty, but in other cases, everyone might agree that it tastes awful! That's okay. Try something else the next time. Also, consider throwing a "protein shake party" for your loved one and other family members. Protein shakes come in many different varieties, and, in this way, you can help your loved one identify the tastiest ones. Protein shakes are very healthy as well as good energy boosters. Other family members may find that they, too, are protein-shake fans.

In short, try to help your loved one make her new eating plan and food preparation as fun as possible and, at times, a family activity. With strategies like this, we often find everyone in the family more conscious of mindful eating and healthier in the process. Although your loved one has a much more limited range of choices and amounts, you'll be surprised by the variety of foods she is still able to eat, as well as the creativity that emerges in preparing them.

Be Positive and Supportive

There will likely be times when your loved one experiences and expresses difficulty, frustration, or disappointment with her new eating plan. This can result in noncompliance with the new program, often resulting in eating the wrong foods, the wrong quantities, insufficient water or nutrient intake, and insufficient exercise. This is normal. When this happens, be supportive of her feelings. Nagging, complaining, and being negative in response to your loved one's feelings can lead to stress, which is often a trigger for even more dysfunctional eating. (See the following section, "Keep Stress Levels Low.") At this time, she needs positive support in order to offset past negativity associated with food and to get back on track as soon as possible. Most important, know that being supportive does not mean taking charge of what your loved one should or should not eat. This is her program, not yours; nagging—including excessive suggestions or directions—can be harmful.

If you truly believe that your loved one is eating in a manner that will seriously injure her health and your interventions do not help, consider making a confidential call to the surgeon's office for advice.

Keep Stress Levels Low

We live in a stressful world, and there's only so much we can do about it. For many of us, stress has become such a part of our lives that it's taken for granted; we continue to push on with too many demands and too little time. Stress can negatively affect the immune system, cognition, and overall function. Most important, it can also be a powerful trigger for overeating, particularly foods that are high in carbohydrates, fat, and calories. These foods may provide a temporary relief from stress, in part by elevating mood and inducing a feeling of relaxation. On the downside, these foods also cause weight gain and are not part of your loved one's new eating plan.

It's essential that you, other friends, and family members make a concentrated effort to reduce the stress in your loved one's life as well as your own, especially now. Try to keep things simple and in perspective. Review the issues at hand together to decide their importance. If something is relatively unimportant—even if you might have stressed about it in the past—practice letting it go. For example, if something doesn't get done right away, take comfort in the fact that unfinished business is the norm for a lot of people. At times you might want to write a to-do list with your loved one, and then, when the tasks are completed, tear it up together! Sometimes, you might want to tear it up even when they are not completed. Always keep in mind that the most important thing right now is your loved one's long-term health.

Aside from everyday stress, your loved one may be stressed because of her new dietary limitations. It's likely that she turned to certain foods to relieve her stress and now no longer has that outlet. It's important that you understand this and be sympathetic, fully supportive, and non-judgmental while your loved one works through this. In the meantime, try to make mealtimes a pleasant experience. You can do this by using pretty table settings, playing soft background music, lighting candles, placing a vase of flowers in the center of the table, or moving meals to a new place in the house every once in a while. Make mealtimes a time to be together. Avoid discussing problems or sensitive issues at the table. Instead, relax and talk about pleasant things, including humorous events of the day or wonderful plans for the future. Save more serious discussion for later. Some couples use an hour or two after dinner to talk about sensitive issues or problems. Also, avoid distractions like watching TV during meals—this often leads to increased eating, usually without awareness.

While it makes sense for mealtimes to be stress free and relaxing, your loved one will need to find other ways to relieve stress. If you put your heads together, you can come up with some creative ideas. Some simple stress-relievers include a walk outside in nature, a bubble bath, and a foot massage.

Another significant source of stress for your loved one are the many changes rapidly taking place in her body and life. As a result of these changes, she may find that people react to her differently than they did before. Your loved one is not exaggerating or imagining this. This does happen and it can be very upsetting. It often brings out a wide range of often confusing and very stressful feelings. Encourage your loved one to talk about what feelings come from this new experience and listen without judgment or surprise. Try to be especially sensitive to these issues as well as the accompanying physical and emotional needs. Communication is the key. Spend as much time as you can talking and listening. Express your thoughts, ask what you can do to help, and consider asking questions rather than making absolute statements.

It's also normal for you to feel stressed by all the changes that are going on around you. You've been through a highly stressful pre-surgical and post-surgical experience along with your loved one. Changes are also occurring in your life and in your relationship with each other. Don't allow yourself to be thrown off base by the changes. You know to expect them. And try not to be hard on yourself if you worry about things, if you become jealous or insecure, or if you feel anger or fear. To make this time as stress free as possible for everyone, you need to be honest with yourself about what you're feeling and openly discuss these feelings with your loved one in a gentle manner. Like your loved one, you can also talk to a trusted friend. Keeping your negative feelings inside may make them grow, leading to anger, insecurity, misunderstanding, distrust, and—in the worst case—actions you may later regret. Only by sharing your concerns and feelings will you find positive solutions and, in some cases, realize that some of your concerns are groundless, meaningless, or easily resolved.

Share in the Positive Changes

As mentioned above, your loved one will be going through many changes. Some of these changes may include new relationships with people and new activities that will help take the place of her past relationship with food. If your loved one is like many of our patients, she may have participated in few outside activities and had more limited relationships. So, when she starts doing more and meeting new people, you might find yourself a bit jealous at first. Understand that it's important for your loved one to develop new, healthy friendships. Make an effort to get to know some of the new people in your loved one's life. Also, try to participate together in these new activities as often as possible. New people and new adventures can make both of your lives more exciting and fulfilling.

HOW TO MAKE LIFE A LITTLE "SWEETER" FOR YOUR LOVED ONE

We applaud you for having read this far and for having taken part in your loved one's journey toward the ultimate destination of a lifetime of health. Now, it's time for dessert—but our dessert has nothing to do with food. The main ingredients in all of our sweets are humor, spontaneity, creativity, and love. Like any good dessert, we urge you to modify the recipes and add your own ingredients. You'll find yourself creating new, exciting, and unique "desserts" for your loved one. Be sure to involve all willing participants in the "cooking" process, especially children who love this sort of thing.

So, if not an edible dessert, what kind of dessert are we talking about? Our sweets are activities and tasks that your loved one can "nibble" on when food cravings become unbearable and stress has taken a firm hold. Cravings come and go like waves; the peak lasts only about ten to fifteen minutes, coming on strong, lessening, and then eventually passing. The time in between is the danger zone. During this time, she needs something to beat the craving. It's hard to pull ideas out of the air, so this is where you and other caring friends and family members come in. Help your loved one create an "Emergency Kit"— a shoebox-sized box—that you will help fill with non-food-related activities and tasks. When your loved one is feeling the urge to eat, she can pick one of the ideas out of the box to focus on something, anything, except food. Food cravings are very much like fires that need to be put out. Reaching into the box to find something to do other than eat is like pulling the lever on the fire alarm in emergency situations.

The following sections discuss some helpful ideas for how to go about making the kit as well as some ideas for what to place inside it.

Making an Emergency Kit

Gather several friends and family members, including your loved one of course, around the kitchen table, not for eating but for creating. Start with a small box; a shoebox is the perfect size. Have plenty of index cards, colored pencils, and fine-tipped markers and perhaps various stickers on hand. Cover the box with construction paper, brown paper, or wrapping paper as if you were wrapping a present, but wrap the top and bottom of the box separately so that it can be opened and closed. If you use unprinted paper, you can decorate it however you'd like.

Once the box has been prepared, give everyone several index cards and then brainstorm about different things you can write on the index cards. Since your loved one is a unique individual, you'll need to tailor the "recipes" you put in the kit to suit her needs. The following sections should help you get started, but remember to come up with your own ideas too. The more goodies there are to choose from, the better.

Things to Include in the Emergency Kit

The activities your group comes up with should be centered on things that do not involve food. For example, if your loved one reaches into the box and pulls out an index card that reads something funny like "run around the house with the dog" or "brush and floss your teeth," the task would take her away from the kitchen and into other parts of the house that are usually food-free. Making the task fun is a real key. Activities such as these provide enough time for that urge to eat to have peaked and then settle down.

Exercise is also a good activity to include in the kit. Don't be too general though. Include several different types of exercises on different index cards. One can be "take a walk around the block or down the street" or "ride the stationary bike for fifteen minutes." You should be able to come up with a lot of different exercises to keep things interesting. Add some cards that appeal to the senses—take a bubble bath, spray on perfume, smell a flower, buy something very colorful, use a new shade of nailpolish. Try to avoid including activities that your loved one associates with eating. For example, if she is used to eating and watching television at the same time, don't include a card that says "watch a TV show." You may want to use a different colored index cards, such as pink or blue in place of the standard white, for those activities your loved one finds most helpful. This will make it easier to pluck them out of the pile when the urge to eat is particularly powerful.

You'll probably want to include some index cards with activities that involve leaving the home. For example, Katie lives in a studio apartment. The bed and the kitchen are side by side. Katie can actually reach food from her bed! Obviously, her "Emergency Kit" must center on getting her out of the house. Some ideas for getting out of the house—when time permits of course—include visiting a friend, going to a museum or to a movie, taking a walk in nature, and window-shopping. You and your group can probably come up with a lot more.

Also, some of the index cards can include things that need to be done around the house. For example, reorganize a dresser drawer or a closet, give the dog a bath, replace missing buttons, repot plants, weed the garden, and so on. Some pleasant distractions include making a phone call to a friend, family member, or support group member; writing a letter or an essay; drawing, painting, or coloring; and playing a musical instrument. Also include personal-care activities, like rubbing on body lotion, exercising, showering, and experimenting with makeup. Other activities can involve other people, too—for example, playing a board game or a game of tennis or Ping-Pong and asking for a hand or neck massage from a good friend. The activities you and the others come up with are limited only by your imagination. Keep in mind that cards can be added to the kit whenever the creative urge hits.

WHEN WISHES COME TRUE FOR THE HOLIDAYS

Holidays and special days such as birthdays are a time of celebration. In addition to the special occasion being celebrated, also use these days to celebrate your loved one's health and all the positive changes she has experienced. Go ahead and make any day a special day if your loved one needs a pick-me-up. Special days often involve giving people you love and care about special gifts. On these days, you can give your loved one "wish-come-true" gifts. These gifts will serve as visible reminders of all of the things your loved one has to be grateful for in a very creative and fun way. Once again, be sure to involve kids in this activity.

Make a list of all the things your loved one has accomplished since her surgery (see the list below for some help). Then, write some of these things on brightly colored paper or other items, such as holiday decorations. Make sure each "granted wish" is highly visible and placed where it can be easily seen for at least a week. When your loved one looks at these granted wishes, she will be reminded that she is a true hero for having had the surgery, taking the risks, and bravely hanging in there. She will also be reminded of just how much she is loved, as well as all the wonderful changes the surgery has made possible for the whole family. Here are some ideas for your wish-come-true messages:

- You fit comfortably in chairs—at home, in the movie theater, on the train, and even in small cars!

- Your "new" lap is just the right size for a child!

- You can bend down from your waist to pick up something you dropped!

- You don't need your diabetes medication anymore!

- You feel great!

- You bask in the glow of compliments from others!

- You can exercise longer!

- You don't need a seat-belt extender on an airplane!

- You glide right through turnstiles!

- You can buy your clothes "off the rack"!

- You've discovered new body parts—like collarbones and hips!

- You've got lots of energy to do more than you ever thought you could!

- You like yourself!

- You feel good about yourself!

- You are even more attractive to others!

- You got that job, raise, or promotion you've always wanted!

- You are so much healthier!

- You have hope for an even better future!

These are just some examples. You can probably come up with a lot more. Encourage your loved one to enjoy her bragging rights! Day by day, she is getting stronger and healthier. That is a truly great gift. There will be plenty to celebrate and be grateful for on the holidays, this year and every year!

CONCLUSION

In this chapter, you learned that there is much you can do to help your loved one recover after surgery and to stay on track with her eating plan, even during the toughest of times. It's wonderful that she has you to count on. You should be very proud of yourself! We have enjoyed sharing a part of the journey with you. All the best!

$\mathscr{C}$ONCLUSION

If you've had weight-loss surgery, we consider you a hero! You've made a valiant effort to improve your health and well-being and to live longer for the sake of yourself as well as many others. You are well on your way to renewed health and increasing happiness. Congratulations! But remember, the hardest work begins after surgery. You must make a lifelong commitment to your new way of life. It will be mostly up to you how much weight you lose and how much you keep off in the coming years. As you know, you'll need to make a lot of changes, but the rewards are well worth it and will be far greater than the effort you make. With your new skills and increased confidence, you *will* succeed. Thank you for allowing us to share in your very special journey.

If you have not yet made up your mind, you now have sufficient facts upon which to base a well-informed decision. This final decision must, of course, rest with you, since you will be undergoing the risk, pain, and expense of weight-loss surgery. Input from your family, friends, and caregivers can be a great help to you while you are trying to make your decision. Also, during the decision-making process, think about the patients' stories you read in this book as well as others like them. These people were once very much like you are now. You'll be glad to know that all of the people mentioned in this book have successfully given themselves a second chance to experience life and are currently making the best of it.

Some people promise themselves that, if they fail in their next weight-loss effort, they'll have the surgery. Some follow through on this promise, and some do not. In this country, we are free to make our own decisions and do so. In many instances, however, tragedy strikes—we have found that many more people die as a result of not having weight-loss surgery than those who die from surgical complications—about three times as many people. And, as for success with non-surgical weight-loss methods, you will have learned from reading this book that the chances of success are about 2 percent at best. Not many people would accept those terrible odds in treating their high blood pressure, cancer, or heart disease if they had another option, which most do. However, we are all "experts" at eating and, therefore, at dieting, and we can sometimes fool ourselves into thinking that we know best and that the "next treatment" will, and must, work. Unfortunately, it rarely, if ever, does.

Clearly, the choice is yours. However, we wish you well, and you will remain in our thoughts and prayers that you are guided toward the most appropriate course for you. Please allow us to sincerely wish you and yours all the best in your journey and struggle to win the war on obesity!

GLOSSARY

Atelectasis. A condition in which the tiny air sacs—called the *alveoli*—in the lungs collapse or become filled with fluid. It commonly occurs following surgery and anesthesia on morbidly obese patients, particularly at the base of the lungs. The use of the incentive spirometer is intended to prevent or treat this condition that may, otherwise, progress to pneumonia.

Band migration. A potential complication of gastric banding that occurs when part of the stomach wall "moves," or migrates, usually inside, through the band. Also called *band displacement*.

Bariatric. Refers to the branch of medicine that deals with the causes, management, research, and prevention of overweight and obesity. The term is derived from the Greek words *baros*, meaning "heavy, and *iatros*, meaning "physician."

Bariatric physician. A physician who specializes in weight-loss management.

Bariatric surgeon. A fully qualified general surgeon who specializes in weight-loss surgery—also called *bariatric surgery*—for the morbidly obese.

Body mass index (BMI). A measure of body fat based on height and weight, which is calculated by dividing weight in kilograms by height in meters squared. The BMI is strongly correlated with body-fat content—that is, the higher the BMI, the higher the likelihood of an increased percentage in total body fat.

Bronchitis. Inflammation of the airways leading to the lungs.

Carcinogens. Cancer-causing substances.

Cardiologist. A heart specialist.

Central sleep apnea. A condition in which part(s) of the brain fail to properly pace breathing during sleep. It may occur together with obstructive sleep apnea. *See also* Obstructive sleep apnea.

Cholecystectomy. Surgical removal of the gallbladder. This procedure is sometimes performed during weight-loss surgery.

Cholecystitis. Inflammation of the gallbladder.

Cirrhosis. Scarring of the liver of varying degree, sometimes expressed as "mild," "moderate," or "severe."

Comorbidities. A group of medical, physical, psychological, social, and economic conditions or illnesses that often occur wth, or get worse with, the development, presence, or progression of obesity.

Coronary artery disease (CAD). A disease in which the arteries that supply blood to the heart muscles are narrowed. When this narrowing becomes severe enough, an individual with CAD may have a heart attack, chest pain (angina), irregular heartbeats, and possibly die.

Cough pillow. A firm pillow, often used following weight-loss surgery, that is pressed over the front of the abdomen to help reduce pain while coughing.

CPAP machine. A device used to treat sleep apnea by helping to "splint" the airways open with pressure; CPAP stands for "continuous positive airway pressure."

Creatinine. A muscle breakdown product, the levels of which are normally quite constant day to day. Creatinine is normally filtered from the blood by the kidneys. Serum creatinine is a measure of kidney (renal) function. In kidney failure, serum creatinine levels will rise.

Deep venous thrombosis. A blood clot that most often forms in the deep veins of the legs, thighs, or pelvis.

Dermatitis. A general term for inflammation of the skin.

Dumping syndrome. A condition in which food and/or liquid nutrients pass too quickly into or through the small intestines; it has been known to occur, to a varying extent, in up to half of the patients who have had gastric bypass surgery. It is most often triggered by eating food that contains a high amount of sugar. It may produce symptoms such as diarrhea, faintness, dizziness, weakness, abdominal pain, sweating, and rapid heart rate with or without an extremely urgent need to have a bowel movement. The usual treatment for this condition includes dietary changes and medication, although in rare cases, revision or reversal of bariatric surgery may be considered.

Echocardiogram. A non-invasive test in which an instrument emitting sound waves produces images of the heart on a monitor. It can image normal and abnormal heart valves and heart-wall thickness, as well as possible fluid in the pericardial sac surrounding the heart.

Edema. Swelling caused by the excessive collection of fluid in the tissues, skin, or organs. It may occur rapidly or slowly. It is described as *pitting edema* when five seconds of finger pressure against a swollen area such as the ankle leaves an indentation that remains for a while and then slowly refills. Lower extremity edema is often found in morbidly obese people.

Endorphins. Chemicals in the brain that may produce positive moods.

Endoscopy. The use of a long, flexible, lighted tube for examining the inside of certain parts of the body, such as the stomach and colon.

Endotracheal tube. An tube inserted into the trachea through the mouth to help control and assist breathing.

End-stage obesity syndrome (ESOS). A life-threatening condition in which a morbidly obese or super-morbidly obese person is experiencing failure of one or more organs and is expected to survive no more than weeks or months.

Enema. An injection of liquid—with or without medication—into the large intestine through the anus.

Foley catheter. A thin tube inserted into the bladder to keep it empty of urine; it is usually attached to a tube and collecting bag into which urine empties, often to assess the volume of urine output.

Gastritis. Inflammation of the stomach.

Gastroesophageal reflux disease (GERD). A condition that occurs when the ring of muscle at the bottom of the esophagus—called the *lower esophageal sphincter*—does not function properly, or close, allowing the acid and other stomach contents to reflux, or leak, backward into the esophagus. The acid causes the lining of the esophagus to become irritated, which, in turn, produces a burning feeling in the front of the chest, called *heartburn,* or the throat. Chest pain, hoarseness, difficulty swallowing, dry coughing, or food sticking in the throat may also occur with or without heartburn. To be referred to as GERD, these symptoms must occur more than two or three times a week.

Gastrostomy tube (G-tube). A drainage tube placed into the stomach through the abdominal wall to drain stomach contents after surgery. It may also be used to administer liquefied medications, food, supplements, or liquids when the patient has difficulty taking them by mouth. In weight-loss surgery patients, the G-tube is placed into the bypassed stomach.

Gout. A disorder in which uric acid crystals deposit in and around joints, causing pain and arthritis. Its presence may be determined by obtaining elevated levels of uric acid in the blood.

Heel spur. A painful growth of bone on the underside of the heel bone that can be irritated by walking.

Helicobacter pylori. A bacteria that can infect the stomach and may cause ulcers.

Hiatus hernia. A condition in which the esophageal hiatus, or opening, of the diaphragm becomes abnormally widened, thereby allowing the upper part or all of the stomach to protrude through it. It may result in symptoms of GERD. *See aslo* Gastroesophagel reflux disease.

Hiatal herniorrhaphy. Surgical repair of a hiatus hernia. This procedure may be performed during weight-loss surgery.

Hirsutism. Excess facial and/or other body hair.

Hypersomnolence. Excessive sleepiness.

Hypertension. High blood pressure.

Incarceration. Entrapment, or imprisonment, of the contents of a hernia.

Incentive spirometer. An apparatus used to encourage the user to produce deep breathing and coughing, especially following surgery. Also called an *inspirometer.*

Insulin. A hormone produced by the pancreas that, among its many other functions, helps move glucose from the blood into muscle cells and other tissues.

Intravenous hyperalimentation (IVH). A method of providing all the nutrients necessary for sustained life directly into a patient's body through a large vein when that individual cannot, will not, or should not eat for days, months, or years.

Locked bowels. A lay term for a condition in which the intestine is kinked or otherwise twisted, preventing food, liquid, or digestive juices from passing downward to the colon. This condition may be associated with poor or absent blood supply to a portion(s) of the bowel that may result in damage or death of a bowel segment(s) and be a reason for emergency abdominal surgery. Also called *small bowel obstruction.*

Malabsorption. Impaired absorption of nutrients by the small intestine.

Morbid obesity. A condition in which a person is 100-plus pounds over ideal body weight, has a BMI of 35 to 39.9 with comorbidities, or a BMI of 40 or higher without comorbidities.

Nasogastric (NG) tube. A flexible plastic tube inserted through the nose and into the stomach that is usually used to suction out the contents of the stomach. It may also be used to provide tube feeding of liquids, nutrients, or liquified medications.

Obesity. A lifelong, progressive, life-threatening, genetically related disease of excessive fat storage with five main comorbidities; these are medical, psychological, social, physical, and economic.

Obesity-hypoventilation syndrome. A condition thought to arise from a combination of inadequate lung expansion due to obesity and a defect in the control of breathing by the brain. This results in abnormally high levels of carbon dioxide along with low oxygen levels in the blood. People with this condition sleep poorly, are chronically tired, often fall asleep during normal waking hours, become short of breath after minimal exertion, and may have a bluish discoloration of the skin, lips, or fingernails. It often occurs together with obstructive sleep apnea. Also called *Pickwickian syndrome.*

Obstructive sleep apnea. A condition in which the airway intermittently becomes completely or partially obstructed during sleep, sometimes occurring more than one hundred times an hour. Affected people typically snore loudly, experience extremely restless sleep, have low blood oxygen levels, experience daytime sleepiness, feel as tired upon awaking as they did when going to sleep, have high blood pressure, and suffer from morning headaches. Their neck circumference is usually very large. This condition is most appropriately diagnosed by use of polysomnography.

Polysomnography. A test that measures one's breathing and other vital signs, electrical signals from the heart, muscle activity, brainwaves, and oxygen in the blood during sleep to identify possible breathing or other sleep-related disorders.

Pseudotumor cerebri. A disorder that involves abnormally elevated pressure in the fluid surrounding the brain and spinal cord that may be associated with severe headaches and reduced vision, leading to possible blindness and paralysis of one of the external eye muscles.

Pulmonary edema. Edema that occurs in the lungs. *See also* Edema.

Pulmonary embolism. A blood clot in the lungs that usually arises elsewhere, most frequently traveling from the deep veins in the legs, thighs, or pelvis.

Pulmonologist. A lung specialist.

Pylorus. The muscular valve at the bottom of the stomach.

Restless leg syndrome. A nervous system disorder associated with unpleasant leg, thigh, foot, or arm sensations—tingling, pins and needles, burning, aching, and jitteriness—while sitting or lying down. These symptoms usually improve, or are relieved, by moving the affected part. When frequent limb movements occur during sleep, this condition is also known as *periodic movement limb disorder;* it may interfere with nighttime sleep, cause drowsiness and fatigue during the day, and is often found in people with obstructive sleep apnea.

Serotonin. A chemical in the brain and other nerves thought to be associated with pleasure. Deficiency may be associated with depression.

Sleep apnea. *See* Central sleep apnea; Obstructive sleep apnea.

Small bowel obstruction. *See* Locked bowels.

Sonogram. An image produced by sound waves passing through part of the body's internal structures.

Stoma. When applied to weight-loss surgery, this term is most commonly used for the point of exit from the stomach pouch into the lower stomach or small intestine.

Super-morbid obesity. A condition in which a person is usually 2.25 times ideal body weight or has a BMI of 50 or more.

Tubal ligation. A surgical procedure in which the fallopian tubes are surgically tied off and divided in order to prevent pregnancy.

Tummy tuck. A lay term for a surgical procedure in which excess skin and fat (the "pannus" or "panniculus") is removed from the lower abdomen; also called an *abdominoplasty*. This surgery usually involves the removal, or reimplantation, of the umbilicus.

Umbilicus. A medical term for the belly button.

Umbilical hernia. A form of ventral hernia that occurs at the umbilicus. *See also* Ventral hernia; Umbilicus.

Urinary stress incontinence. Impairment or loss of bladder control, usually resulting from coughing, sneezing, straining, or any other activity that elevates pressure within the abdominal cavity and the organs contained within it, including the bladder.

Varicose veins. Enlarged, often tortuous, veins in the lower extremities that appear most prominently while standing. They are usually associated with incompetent, or non-functioning, valves in the vein. This condition may be associated with swollen feet, ankles, or legs and, in severe cases, leg ulceration may occur.

Ventilator. A machine to help assist with, or control, breathing.

Ventral hernia. A weakness or defect of the abdominal wall through which tissues inside the abdominal cavity protrude abnormally.

Waterbrash. Bitter-tasting, acidic, clear liquid from the stomach that runs up into the mouth; a symptom of hiatus hernia.

RESOURCES

American Obesity Association
1250 24th Street, NW, Suite 300
Washington, DC 20037
Phone: 202-776-7711
Fax: 202-776-7712
Website: www.obesity.org

**American Society for Bariatric
  Surgery (ASBS)**
100 SW 75th Street, Suite 201
Gainesville, FL 32607
Phone: 352-331-4900
Fax: 352-331-4975
E-mail: info@asbs.org
Website: www.asbs.org

**International Association of
  Eating Disorder Professionals
  (IAEDP)**
P.O. Box 1295
Pekin, IL 61555-1295
Phone: 800-800-8126
Fax: 309-346-2874
Website: www.iaedp.com

Obesity Help, Inc.
Website: www.obesityhelp.com/
  morbidobesity/

*A comprehensive obesity-related
website that offers support, helpful
information, and various resource
tools.*

Web MD
Website: www.webmd.com

*Provides general medical information.
For a list of sponsored links relating
to weight-loss surgery, type
BARIATRIC SURGERY into the search
bar on Web MD's homepage.*

WLS Help
Website: www.wlshelp.com

*Provides the latest news and
information on the surgical
treatment of obesity.*

REFERENCES

Buchwald H. "Consensus Conference Statement: Bariatric surgery for morbid obesity: health implications for patients, health professionals, and third-party payers." *J Am Coll Surg* 2005;200:593–604.

Deitel, Mervyn (Ed.) and Cowan, George. *Update: Surgery for the Morbidly Obese Patient.* Toronto: FD-Communications, 2000.

Drenick, E. J., Bale, G. S., Seltzer F., and Johnson, D. G. "Excessive mortality and causes of death in morbidly obese men," *The Journal of the American Medical Association,* Vol. 243, No. 5, February 1, 1980.

Gastrointestinal Surgery for Severe Obesity. NIH Consensus Statement 1991 Mar 25–27;9(1):1–20.

$\mathcal{A}$BOUT
THE AUTHORS

Merle Cantor Goldberg, LCSW, DSCW, CEDS, received a diplomate in clinical social work from the University of Maryland, and has specialized in treating eating disorders for over thirty-five years. Over this period, she has served as a training leader for the International Association of Eating Disorders. Currently the Executive Director of Associates in Psychotherapy, she has appeared on many radio and television shows and is a highly sought-after lecturer. Ms. Goldberg's articles have been published in numerous newspapers and magazines, and she is the co-author of *My Thin Excuse* and *The Human Circle*.

George Cowan, Jr., MD, is a Professor of Surgery at the University of Tennessee Medical School. He has been President of the American College of Nutrition, and Director for the Masters' Course of the American Society for Bariatric Surgery. In addition, he is cofounder of the medical journal *Obesity Surgery*, and founder of the International Federation for the Surgery of Obesity. Dr. Cowan is the co-editor/co-author of three textbooks for surgeons on obesity surgery, and the author of over 300 medical and scientific articles. He lectures to professional groups throughout the world.

William Y. Marcus, MD, is a retired Clinical Assistant Professor of Surgery at George Washington University Medical School. Dr. Marcus has over four decades of surgical experience, including twenty years specializing in bariatric surgery. He is founder and leader of a large, self-help obesity surgery-support group, serving hundreds of pre-op and post-op patients throughout the greater Washington, DC area.

$\mathcal{I}$NDEX

Abdomen, swollen, 148, 164
Abdominal binder, 142–143
Abdominal crunches, 178
Abdominal drain, 138
Abdominal pain
    persistent, 193–194
    severe, 164
Abdominal sonogram, 99
Abdominoplasty. *See* Tummy tuck.
Acetaminophen, 162
Actigall, 171
Adjustable gastric banding (AGB),
    40–42
    possible complications of, 42
Advil, 162
Aerobic exercise, 177
AGB. *See* Adjustable gastric
    banding.
Age, qualifying for surgery and,
    22–23
AIDS, as a disqualifier for surgery, 27
Albumin, 188
Alcohol consumption
    after surgery, 170–171
    qualifying for surgery and, 26
    questions about, 97
Alcohol in medication, 162

Alcoholics, 26
Aleve, 162
Alimentary limb. *See* Food limb.
Alka-Seltzer, 162
American Board of Surgery, 59
American Society for Bariatric
    Surgery (ASBS), 19, 21, 57–58, 76
    guidelines for surgery, 19, 20, 21,
    22, 24
    Surgical Review Corporation, 58
Anacin-3, 162
Anaerobic exercise, 177
Anesthesia
    receiving, 129
    waking up from, 131
Anesthesiologist, consultation with,
    102–103
Anger, caution about, 200
Antibiotics, taking prior to surgery,
    125
Antidepressants, 146
Antioxidants, cancer risk and, 10
Antiseptic soap, washing with, 125
Arterial blood gases (ABG) testing.
    See Blood work.
Arterial line, 140
Artificial sweeteners, 176

ASBS. *See* American Society for Bariatric Surgery.
Ascriptin, 162
Aspirin, 162
Atelectasis, 119
Audiotapes, motivational. *See* Positive-reinforcement messages.
Awake intubation, 129

Band displacement, 42
Band inflation, 40
Band migration. *See* Band displacement.
Banded gastric bypass, 46
Bariatric surgeon. *See* Weight-loss surgeon.
Bariatric surgery. *See* Weight-loss surgery.
Barium sulfate, 101
Basic metabolic panel (BMP). *See* Blood work.
Beck Depression Inventory, 106
Bed
    getting out of, after surgery, 142–143
    hospital, 115
    technique for getting out of, 120
Beverage(s)
    carbonated. *See* Carbonated beverages.
    choices, 170
    high-calorie, 173
    See also Drinking; Fluid intake.
Bilevel positive airway pressure (BiPAP) machine. *See* BiPAP machine.
Biliopancreatic diversion (BPD), 46–47
Biliopancreatic limb. *See* Digestive-juice limb.

Bills, paying, during hospital stay, 117
Binder, abdominal. *See* Abdominal binder.
Binder (three-ring), as a presurgical gift, 234
Bingeing, 199. *See also* Overeating, compulsive.
BiPAP machine, 102
Birth control, 160–161
Bladder control, loss of. *See* Urinary stress incontinence.
Bleeding, controlling postsurgical, 147
Bloating, narcotics and, 134
Blood
    clots. *See* Blood clot(s).
    in the stool, 164
    tests. *See* Blood work.
    vomiting, 164
Blood clot(s)
    and excessive risk, 26
    prevention, 119, 141, 146–147
Blood donations, avoiding, 163
Blood donors, verifying arrangements with, 112
Blood work
    periodic, 192
    postsurgical, 142
    presurgical, 98–99, 124–125
Blood-thinning medication, 146
BMI. *See* Body mass index.
Body cues, distorted. *See* Body image, distortion.
Body image
    becoming grounded to improve, 214
    challenges to, 206
    creating new, 210–213
    development of, 209
    distortion, 208, 209, 213

issues concerning, 207–213
Body mass index (BMI), 20–21
Body weight, qualifying for surgery
and, 20–21
Body-fat analysis, 180
Body-lift surgery. *See* Plastic surgery.
Boots, inflatable. *See* Inflatable
boots.
Bowel movements, keeping tracking
of, 152. *See also* Stool.
BPD. *See* Biliopancreatic diversion.
BPD-DS. *See* BPD-duodenal switch.
BPD-duodenal switch (BPD-DS), 47
Breast cancer. *See* Cancer, in the
morbidly obese.
Breathing difficulties, 9, 164
Breathing exercises. *See* Deep-
breathing exercises.
Breathing tests, 101–102
Bufferin, 162
Bulge, protruding, 165
Bypassed stomach, concerns about,
193

CAD. *See* Coronary artery disease.
Caffeine consumption, effects of, 170
Calcium supplements, 174
Calel-D, 174
Caloric intake, 167–168, 186–188
Calorie balance, 188
Caltrate 600, 174
Cancer, in the morbidly obese, 9–10
Carbon dioxide, 166
Carbonated beverages, 149–150. *See
also* Fluid intake, cautions about.
Care, need for round-the-clock, 247
Central sleep apnea, 15
Checklists
for going home, 153
for presurgical preparations, 122
Chenodeoxycholic acid, 52

Chest pain, 164
Children
caring for, postsurgically, 248–249
confirming arrangements for care,
115–116
reassuring after surgery, 244
reassuring before surgery,
239–241
weight-loss surgery in, 22
Chills, 164
Cholecystectomy. *See* Gallbladder
removal.
Cholecystitis, 11
Cholesterol. *See* High-density
lipoprotein (HDL); Low-density
lipoprotein (LDL).
Climbing stairs. *See* Stair climbing,
during recovery.
Clothing, 115, 157–158
Cold, reporting prior to surgery, 124
Comfort, providing, 248
Common limb, 44, 45, 47, 63, 152
Comorbidities, 5
insurance coverage and, 23
list of, 8
qualifying for surgery and, 23
plastic surgery and, 216
Company, arranging for
postsurgical, 118
Complete blood count (CBC). *See*
Blood work.
Complications, 42, 45, 46, 66, 99, 193,
216
and exercise, 120
and hospital bill, 31, 33
and surgeon's experience, 62
and surgical approaches, 36
eating disorders and, 104
Glucophage and, 113
leg position and, 147
psychological, 106

swollen abdomen and, as a sign of, 148

Compliance with program
long-term, 197–198
postsurgical support and, 80–81

Comprehensive metabolic panel (CMP). *See* Blood work.

Compulsive overeating. *See* Overeating, compulsive.

Confusion, 164

Congestive heart failure, and excessive risk, 26

Constipation, narcotics and, 134

Continued education, postsurgical support and, 80

Continuous positive air pressure (CPAP) machine. *See* CPAP machine.

Coricidin, 162

Coronary artery disease (CAD), 11–12

Cortisone, 162

Cosmetic surgery. *See* Plastic surgery.

Cough pillow, 121, 137

Coughing exercises, 119–120, 137

CPAP machine, 102

CPAP titration study, 102

Cramping pain, severe, 165

Cravings. *See* Food cravings, activities to overcome; Sweet cravings, concerns about.

Creatinine, 192

Crunches, abdominal. *See* Abdominal crunches.

Cyst removal, 54

Dating. *See* Relationship(s), romantic and sexual.

Datril, 162

Deep venous thrombosis, 102

and excessive risk, 26

Deep-breathing exercises, 119–120, 125, 137, 157

Denial of weight-related problems, 27

Deodorant spray, 152

Depression, 23–24, 145–146, 159–162, 250

Diabetes mellitus, 10

Diarrhea
persistent, 193–194
severe, 165

Diet. *See* Eating.

Diet, liquid. *See* Liquid diet, advancing to; Liquids-only diet.

Diet, weight-loss, failure of, 21, 28–29

Digestive-juice limb, 44–45

Dinnerware, smaller, 151

Discharge from the hospital, 152–154
checklist for, 153

DNA damage, and cancer risk, 10

Dolobid, 162

Downtime, being creative with, 205

Drain. *See* Abdominal drain; Subcutaneous drain.

Drainage from wound. *See* Wound drainage.

Drenick, Ernst J., 17

Drinking
and eating, waiting period, 150
avoiding at mealtimes, 169
after surgery, 149
See also Beverages; Fluid intake.

Driving, during recovery, 159

Drug use, as a disqualifier for surgery, 26

Dumping syndrome, 48

Duodenal switch. *See* BPD-duodenal switch.

Eating
and drinking, waiting period, 150
after surgery, 148–152
behavior. *See* Eating habits.
disorders. *See* Eating disorders.
masking feelings by, 199
plan. *See* Eating plan, new.
Eating disorders, 191
assessing for, 104
See also Overeating.
Eating habits
changing, 168
dealing with presurgical, 191
developing proper, 190
family-wide changes and,
251–252
See also Eating plan, new.
Eating out cards. *See* Meal cards.
Eating plan, new, 167–174
help making it work, 250–252
Echocardiogram (EKG), 99–100
Edema, 16–17, 188
EGD. *See*
Esophagogastrodudenoscopy.
EKG. *See* Echocardiogram.
Elastin, 192
Elderly people, weight-loss surgery
in, 22–23
Emergencies
during recovery, 163–166
when to call the surgeon, 164–165
Emergency kit activity, 255–257
Emergency notice card, 166
Emotional abuse, 202
Emotional support for support
person, 241–242
Empirin, 162
Endometrial cancer. *See* Cancer, in
the morbidly obese.
Endorphins, 177
Endotracheal tube, 129

End-stage obesity syndrome (ESOS),
7
Enema, taking prior to surgery, 125,
127
Enlarged esophagus, 42
Enlarged liver, 10
Epidural anesthesia, 136
Esophagogastrodudenoscopy
(EGD), 100
Esophagus, enlarged. *See* Enlarged
esophagus.
ESOS. *See* End-stage obesity
syndrome.
Excedrin, 162
Excessive risks, and qualifying for
surgery, 25–26
Exercise, 205
aerobic, 177
anaerobic, 177
grounding, 214
hydration during, 179
importance of, 193
program. *See* Exercise program.
See also Abdominal crunches;
Coughing exercises; Deep-
breathing exercises; Leg-
pumping exercises; Resistance
training.
Exercise program, 174, 177–181
pointers for, 178–179
help implementing a presurgical,
237–238
Extended gastric bypass (X-GBP),
45–46

Fast food, healthier, 239
Fat, breakdown of, 166
FDA. *See* Food and Drug
Administration.
Fears and doubts, dealing with
postsurgical, 244–245

Feedback, 150, 169
Feelings
 getting professional help to deal
  with, 201
 letting them come, 199–200
 talking about, 200–201
 writing or drawing about, 201
Feldene, 162
Fenfluramine, 100
Fen-phen, 100
Fever, 115
Fioricet, 162
Fiorinal, 162
5-hydroxytryptamine, 189
Flu, reporting prior to surgery, 124
Fluid intake, 176
 cautions about, 170–171
 daily, 168–170
 during exercise, 179
 See also Beverage(s); Drinking.
Fluid pressure on the brain. *See*
 Pseudotumor cerebri.
Fluid retention, 166. *See also* Edema.
Foley catheter, 140–141
Food
 activities to overcome cravings
  for, 255–257
 concerns about limitations
  involving, 198
 easy-to-chew, 175
 feelings and combinations of, 203
 hunger for, dealing with, 189–191
 introducing new, 175
 leftover, 149
 masking feelings by eating, 199
 puréed, 114, 150
 relationship with, 198–199
 reporting accurate intake of, 78
 role of, in self-image, 206
 stress and, 201–203
 to avoid, 173, 176

Food and Drug Administration
 (FDA), 40, 51
Food limb, 43, 44, 45, 47, 48, 63
Food mind, 198
Friends, relationship(s) with old,
 220–222

Gallbladder disease, 11
Gallbladder removal, 52
Gallstones, 11, 99
Gas
 intestinal, 144–145
 pains, technique for preventing,
  144–145
 passing, 144
Gastric banding, 40–42
Gastric bypass (GBP) surgery
 regular, 43–45
 variations, 45–47
Gastric pacemaker, 51
Gastric pouch. *See* Pouch.
Gastroplasty, 38–40
Gastrostomy tube (G-tube), 139
 caring for at home, 158
 insertion of, 51–52
Genetic role in obesity, recognizing,
 29–30
GI series, 100–101
Gifts
 get-well, 240
 "wish-come-true," 257–258
Ginkgo biloba, 113
Glucophage, 113
Gorging, 121, 187, 199. *See also*
 Overeating, compulsive.
Grounding exercise, 214
G-tube. *See* Gastrostomy tube.

H&P. *See* History and physical
 exam.
Hair growth, excess. *See* Hirsutism.

Head hunger, 189
Health, focusing on, 155–163
Health insurance
    comorbidities and coverage, 23
    qualifying for coverage, 31–33
    protocol, 107
    sample letter for, 107–109
Health Insurance Portability &
        Accountability Act (HIPAA) of
        1996, 70
Heart monitor, 139
Heart problems, 11–12
    detecting. *See* Echocardiogram
        (EKG).
Heart rate
    fast, 164
    maximum, 179
    target, 179
Heartburn, 12
Helicobacter pylori, 100
Hepatomegaly. *See* Enlarged liver.
Hiatal herniorrhaphy. *See* Hiatus
        hernia, repair.
Hiatus hernia, 12
    repair, 52–53
High blood pressure. *See*
        Hypertension.
High-density lipoprotein (HDL), 13
Hirsutism, 13
History and physical exam (H&P),
        123–124
Holidays and special occasions,
        planning for, 257–258
Hospital
    bed, arranging for, 115
    checking into the, 126
    discharge from the, 152–154
    help at, from support person, 246
    packing for stay at, 120–121
Hotel reservations, confirming,
        118–119

Housekeeping, prior to surgery, 117
Humor, weight issues and, 207
Hunger, dealing with, 189–191. *See
    also* Food, activities to overcome
    cravings for.
Hypertension, 13–14
Hysterectomy, 54

IAEDP. *See* International Association
        of Eating Disorder Professionals
Ibuprofen, 162
ICU. *See* Intensive-care unit.
Ideal body weight, figuring, 65
Identity, discovering new, 206–207.
        See also Body image.
Ileus, 148
Imminent death, increased
        awareness of, 27–28
INAMED, 40
Incentive spirometer, 119, 125, 137,
        142, 157
Indocin, 162
Infection in wound. *See* Wound
        infection.
Infections, reporting prior to
        surgery, 124
Infertility, 14
Inflatable boots, 141, 146
Information, organizing, 234
Informed consent
        form, 55, 123
        qualifying for surgery and, 24–25
Injection before surgery, 127–128
Insensitive spirometer, 137
Insomnia, 164
Inspirometer. *See* Incentive
        spirometer.
Instructions, willingness to carry out,
        qualifying for surgery and, 25
Intensive care unit (ICU), 130, 131,
        132

International Association of Eating
    Disorder Professionals (IAEDP),
    212
International Classification of
    Diseases, 6, 7
Internet
    finding support on, 88–89, 91–92
    sorting out the good from the bad
        on, 90–91
Intestinal gas, 144–145
Intravenous (IV) fluid tubing, 140
Irritability, 164
Iron. *See* Nutritional supplements.
IV. *See* Intravenous (IV) fluid tubing.

Jaundice, 11

Knowles, Jarol B., 247

Lab tests, 124–125. *See also* Blood
    work.
Lactose intolerance, 150
Laparoscopic bariatric surgery, 36–37
Lap-Band, 40
Lap-Band surgery. *See* Adjustable
    gastric banding.
Last supper. *See* Meals, last "normal."
Last will and testament, updating,
    117–118
Laxative, taking prior to surgery, 125
Leakage, 40, 66
Leftovers, pushing away, 149
Leg, increased swelling in, 164
Leg position, 147
Leg ulcers, 16–17
Leg-pumping exercises, 119–120,
    125, 146, 157
Letter of Medical Necessity, 107
Lifting, 165
    during recovery, 156–157
Liquid diet, advancing to full, 150

Liquids-only diet, 121, 125
Liver biopsy, 53
Liver disease, and excessive risk, 26
Liver, enlarged. *See* Enlarged liver.
Living will, preparing, 117–118
Loading dose, PCA pump and, 135
Locked bowels, 148. *See also* Small
    bowel obstruction, risk of.
Long limb GBP. *See* Extended gastric
    bypass.
Love and affirmation, providing,
    245–246
Low-density lipoprotein (LDL), 13
Lung problems, narcotics and, 134
Lungs, clot in. *See* Pulmonary
    embolism.

Mail and newspapers, placing on
    hold, 116–117
Malabsorptive bariatric surgery,
    42–47
Malnutrition, 27, 45, 46, 47, 48, 64,
    99, 103, 169 188–189
Marriage. *See* Relationship(s), with
    spouse.
Mason, Edward E., 38
Maximum heart rate, 179
Meal cards, 174
Meals
    arrangements for postsurgical,
        113–114
    last "normal," 83, 121–122
    See also Food.
Mealtimes
    making them pleasant, 253
    scheduling, 176
Measurements, taking, 116, 166
Meclomen, 162
Med-Alert card, 166
Medical appointments/visits
    as postsurgical support, 77–80

follow-ups, necessity of, 191–192
H&P, 123–124
initial exam, 98
postsurgical, 181–182
support person and, 234–235
Medical conditions associated with
  obesity. *See* Comorbidities.
Medical history, providing, 96–97
Medications
  blood-thinning, 146
  during recovery, 162–163
  narcotic, 134–135
  prior to surgery, 126
  resuming, 145
  stocking up on postsurgical, 113
  verifying which to take and
    discontinue, 112–113
  See also Pain medication.
Menstrual irregularities, 14
Mental-health specialist,
  consultation with, 105–107
Metcalf, Barbara, 177
Mood swings, support person and,
  249–250
Morbid obesity, 6–7
Motrin, 162
Multidisciplinary team approval,
  23–24
Multivitamins. *See* Nutritional
  supplements.
Muscle, 177
  loss, 180
  versus fat, 166

Nalfon, 162
Naprosyn, 162
Narcotic pain medication. *See* Pain
  medication, narcotic.
Nasogastric (NG) tube, 138
National Institutes of Health (NIH),
  64, 65

Consensus Development
  Conference on Surgery for
  Severe Obesity, 19
Nausea
  after surgery, 145
  persistent, 193–194
NG tube. *See* Nasogastric (NG) tube.
Nibbling, 173
NIH guidelines, 19, 20, 21, 22, 23, 24,
  26, 31, 32
Non-surgical weight-loss methods,
  failure of, 27, 68, 260
Norgesic, 162
Nutrition, postsurgical, 151–152
Nutrition principles, overview of,
  175–176
Nutritional changes, help
  implementing presurgical,
  238–239
Nutritional supplements, 173–174,
  175–176, 188
  stocking up on postsurgical, 113
  verifying which to take and
    discontinue, 112–113
Nutritionist
  consultation with, 103–104
  follow-up with, 176

Obesity
  defined, 5–7
  illnesses associated with. *See*
    Comorbidities.
  odds of dying prematurely and,
    17
Obesity-related health conditions.
  See Comorbidities.
Obstructive sleep apnea, 15
Online support groups. *See* Internet,
  finding support on.
Open bariatric surgery, 36
Operating room

arriving in the, 129
   holding area, 128
   who's who in the, 128
Opinions, dealing with negative,
   236–237
Ovarian cancer. *See* Cancer, in the
   morbidly obese.
Overeating, compulsive, 202–203
   emotional triggers for, 199
Oxygen-delivery device, 137–138
Oxygen-level monitor, 143–144
Oxygen-sensor clip, 139–140

Pacific Laparoscopy, 177
PACU. *See* Post-anesthesia care unit.
Pain
   abdominal, 164, 193–194
   bone, joint, and/or muscle, 9
   increased, 164
   persistent, 193–194
   severe, 164, 165
Pain management
   during recovery, 158–159
   postsurgical, 133–137
Pain medication
   forms of delivery, 135–137
   injections of, 136
   narcotic, 134–135
   non-narcotic, 135
   oral, 136–137
   pump. *See* Patient-controlled
   analgesia (PCA) pump.
Pale skin, 164
Pampering yourself, 204–205
Panadol, 162
Patient-controlled analgesia (PCA)
   pump, 135–136
PCA pump. *See* Patient-controlled
   analgesia (PCA) pump.
Pepto-Bismol, 162
Perception, others, 219–220

Pet care, confirming arrangements
   for, 115–116
Phentermine, 100
Physical activity, increasing for
   exercise, 180
Physical exam, presurgical. *See*
   History and physical exam
   (H&P).
Pill crusher, 114
Plastic surgeon, finding and
   consulting with a, 215–216
Plastic surgery, 213–217
Plateaus, weight loss and, 166–167,
   186–187
Pneumonia prevention, 119
Polysomnogram (PSG), 102
Positive changes, sharing in,
   254–255
Positive imagery. *See* Positive
   thinking.
Positive messages
   listening for, from others, 213
   recording in a journal, 211
Positive self-talk, 212
Positive thinking, 120
Positive-reinforcement messages,
   132–133
Post-anesthesia care unit (PACU),
   130, 131
Posters. *See* Positive-reinforcement
   messages.
Postsurgical support
   continued education, 80
   from friends and family, 84
   help with compliance, 80–81
   medical visits, 77–78
Pouch, 35, 37, 38, 39, 40, 42, 43, 46, 47,
   48, 53, 115, 137, 138, 145, 149, 150,
   163, 169, 170, 175, 186, 187, 189
Predetermination Benefits Letter,
   107

Pregnancy, issues concerning, 25, 160–161
Presurgical preparations, 111–121
  checklist, 122
Presurgical support
  from friends and family, 82–84
  from surgeon's office, 75–77
Presurgical tests and consultations, 98–106
Primary-care physician, the role of, 56–57
ProMod protein supplement, 171
Prostate cancer. *See* Cancer, in the morbidly obese.
Protecting yourself, 204
Protein intake, 171–172, 176, 188–189, 190
  strength training and, 180
  See also Nutrition, postsurgical.
Protein-shake party, 252
Pseudotumor cerebri, 14
PSG. *See* Polysomnogram.
Pulmonary embolism, 26, 66, 102.
  See also Blood clots.
Pulmonary hypertension, and excessive risk, 26
Pulmonologist, visit with, 101–102
Puréed food
  advancing to, 150
  preparing and storing, 114
Pylorus, 47, 52, 139

Quality of life, desire for a better, 28

Rapid breathing, 164
Rapid gastric emptying. *See* Dumping syndrome.
Recovery room, 130, 131
Regurgitation, slight. *See* Feedback.
Rehabilitation center, arranging for a stay at, 118

Relationship(s)
  changes in, after surgery, 70–71
  professional, 228–229
  romantic and sexual, 225–228
  with children, 222–223
  with old friends, 220–222
  with parents, 222
  with spouse, 223–225
Renfrew Center, 207
Resistance training, 166
  muscle groups and, 179–180
Ressler, Adrienne, 207, 208, 209, 211, 212
Restaurant cards. *See* Meal cards.
Resting at home, during recovery, 156
Restrictive bariatric surgery, 37–42
Retractor, pain from, 134
Roux, Cesar, 43
Roux-en-Y gastric bypass. *See* Gastric bypass (GBP) surgery, regular.

Sadness, 164. *See also* Depression.
Sagging skin, concerns about, 192–193. *See also* Skin, loose.
Self-image, challenges to, 206. *See also* Body image.
Senses, elevating your, 205
Seroma, 138
Serotonin, 159–160, 203
Sexual abuse, 202, 227
Sexual activity, during recovery, 159
Shaking, 164
Sick leave, 111–112
Silastic ring gastroplasty (SRG), 38–39
Sipping liquids, after surgery, 149
Skin, loose, 215. *See also* Sagging skin, concerns about.
Sleep apnea, 14–15

central, 15
obstructive, 15
testing for, 102
Sleep study, 102
Sleepiness, excessive, 164
Sleeping arrangements, after
    surgery, 115, 156
Sleeping excessively, 205
Slurring words, 164
Small bowel obstruction, risk of,
    194
Smoking, 97
    in the hospital, 143
Snacking, 168, 176, 187
Specialists, postsurgical visits from,
    142
Spirituality, 204
Staged operation, 48
Stair climbing, during recovery, 156
Step down unit, 132
Stoma, 38, 39, 41, 42
Stomach, bypassed. *See* Bypassed
    stomach, concerns about.
Stomach, message from your. *See*
    Feedback.
Stomach pouch. *See* Pouch.
Stomach stapling, 38
Stool
    blood in the, 164
    frequent and watery, 152
    See also Bowel movements,
    keeping track of.
Stress levels, help reducing, 253–254
Stressors
    reevaluating, 203
    removing, 201–205
Stretching, 178
Subcutaneous drain, 138–139
Substance abuse, as a disqualifier
    for surgery, 26–27
Super-morbid obesity, 7

Supplements. *See* Nutritional
    supplements.
Support, finding
    in your surgeon and staff, 75–81
    in your friends and family,
    81–84
    on the Internet, 88–92
    in a support group, 84–88
Support after surgery, help making
    arrangements for, 239
Support from family/friends, 24,
    81–82
    presurgical, 82–84
    postsurgical, 84
Support group, 57
    attending before initial medical
    visit, 94–95
    company at the, 235
    finding support in, 84–85
    postsurgical support from, 87–88
    presurgical support from, 85–87
    typical happenings at meeting of,
    94–95
Support person
    presurgical tasks for, 233–242
    postsurgical tasks for, 244–258
Surgery. *See* Weight-loss surgery.
Surgical reversal. *See* Weight-loss
    surgery, reversal of.
Surgical staplers, 41
Surgical wound. *See* Wound.
Sweet cravings, concerns about, 189
Sweeteners, artificial. *See* Artificial
    sweeteners.
Swelling in the legs, increased, 164

Temperature, high, 164
Temptation, reducing, 251
Thermometer, 114
Three Factor Eating Questionnaire,
    106

Tolectin, 162
Touch, sense of, 209
Traveling, during recovery, 159
Traveling home, after surgery, 154
Triglycerides, 13
Tryptophan, 203
Tubal ligation, 54
Tummy tuck, 54, 215, 216
Tums antacids, 174
Tylenol, 162
Type-2 diabetes, 10

Ulcers, leg. *See* Leg ulcers.
UNJURY protein supplement, 171
Update: Surgery for the Morbidly Obese Patient (Cowan, et al.), 214–215
Upper gastrointestinal endoscopy, 100–101
Urinary stress incontinence, 15
Utensils, smaller. *See* Dinnerware, smaller.

Vanquish, 162
Varicose veins, 16–17
VBG. *See* Vertical banded gastroplasty.
Venous stasis ulcers. *See* Leg ulcers.
Venous thrombosis, 119
Ventilator, to assist breathing, 130
Ventral hernias, 166
    repair, 53
Vertical banded gastroplasty (VBG), 38–39
Visitors at the hospital, 143
    dealing with, 245
Vomiting
    after surgery, 145
    excessive, 164
    persistent, 193–194
    with blood, 164

Waiting room
    at surgeon's office, 78–79
    during surgery, 128
Walking, 147
    for exercise, 177
    in place, 142
    in water. *See* Water walking.
Wardrobe. *See* Clothing.
Water consumption. *See* Fluid intake.
Water retention, and weight, 166–167
Water walking, 238
Waterbrash, 12
Weakness, 164
Websites, finding reputable. *See* Internet, sorting out the good from the bad on.
Weigh-in, 96
Weighing yourself, 166–167
Weight, mild increase in, 187
Weight and Lifestyle Inventory, 106
Weight fluctuations, 166
Weight gain, and caloric intake, 188
Weight loss
    assessing progress, 166–167
    concern about too much, 186–188
    factors involved in, 187
    leveling off prematurely, 186
    period of, 167
    pitfall, 173
    tracking progress, 116
Weight prejudice, 30–31
Weight-loss attempts, qualifying for surgery and, 21–22
Weight-loss methods, failure of non-surgical, 21, 68, 260
Weight-loss surgeon(s)
    choosing among, 59–66
    experience of, 62, 63
    familiarizing yourself with, 58–59

finding, 57–66
first appointment with, 95–98
learning curve and, 62
locating in your area, 57–58
number of surgeries performed
    by, 62–63
questionnaire for, 60–61
Weight-loss surgery
    and risk of complications, 69
    and risk of death, 68
    avoiding new or experimental,
        63–64
    complications associated with.
        See Complications.
    day of the, 126–130
    death rates associated with, 65–66
    discussing with family, friends,
        and colleagues, 66–72
    discussing with PCP, 56–57
    future alternatives to, 50–51
    help making the decision to have,
        236
    help with the preparations for,
        237–237–241
    in children, 22
    in the elderly, 22–23
    laparoscopic approach to, 36–37
    length of procedure, 63
    malabsorptive. *See* Malabsorptive
        bariatric surgery.
    newer approaches to, 47–49, 51
    open approach to, 36
    procedures commonly performed
        during, 51–54

psychological and emotional
    qualifiers for, 27–31
qualification guidelines, 20–27
restrictive. *See* Restrictive
    bariatric surgery.
reversal of, 194–195
surgical approaches to. *See*
    Laparoscopic bariatric surgery;
    Open bariatric surgery.
weight-loss potential associated
    with, 64–65, 186
Weight-loss-surgery program, help
    complying with, 80–81. *See also*
    Compliance with program.
Weight-loss-surgery support groups.
    See Support group.
Work issues
    approval for extended sick leave,
        111–112
    discussing surgery with boss and
        coworkers, 70–71
    returning to work, 163
    See also Relationships,
        professional.
Wound
    drainage from, 158
    dressings, 141
    increased drainage from, 165
    infection in, 158
    keeping an eye on, 158
    oozing, 164

X-rays, checking progress with,
    147–148